Yoga Heals Your Back

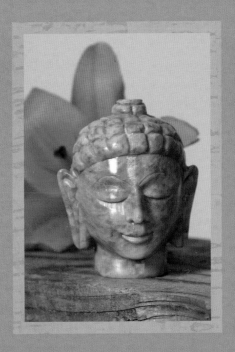

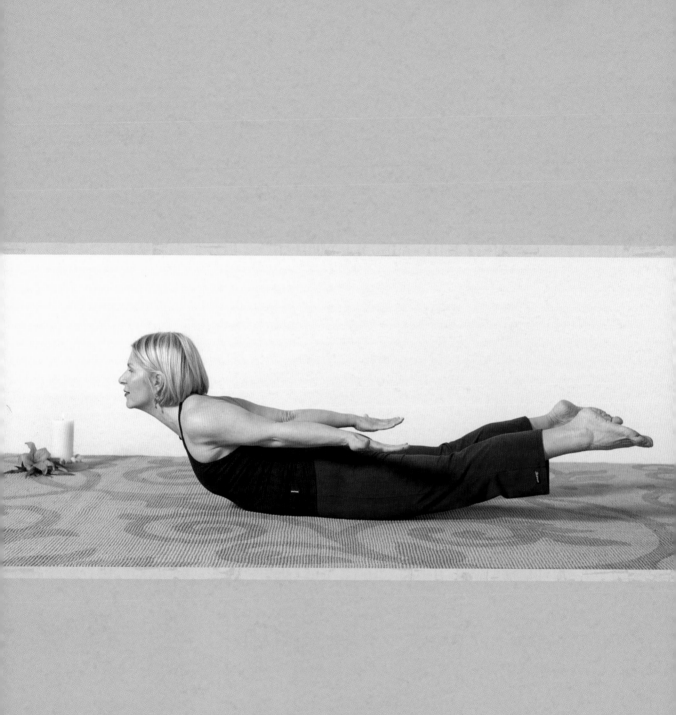

Yoga Heals Your Back

10-Minute Routines That End Back and Neck Pain

R I T A   T R I E G E R

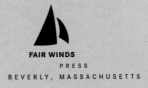

FAIR WINDS
P R E S S
BEVERLY, MASSACHUSETTS

First published in the USA in 2005 by
Fair Winds Press, a member of
Quayside Publishing Group
100 Cummings Center
Suite 406-L
Beverly, MA 01915
www.fairwindspress.com

09   6 7

ISBN-13: 978-1-59233-093-5
ISBN-10: 1-59233-093-2

Library of Congress Cataloging-in-Publication Data available

Book design by Yee Design

Printed and bound in China

The information in this book is for educational purposes only. It is not intended to replace the
advice of a physician or medical practitioner. Please see your health care provider before beginning any new health program.

Dedication

For all of my students who continuously give me beautiful
gifts of inspiration, knowledge, and love.

Namaste

Contents

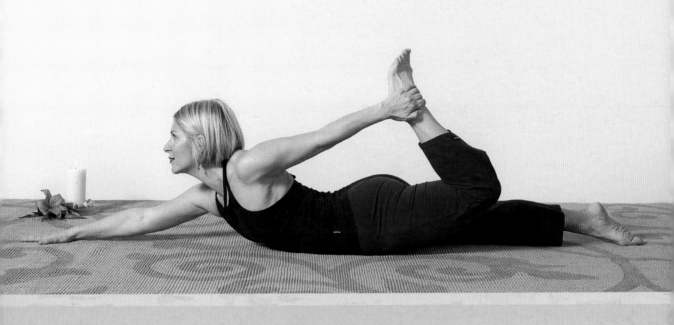

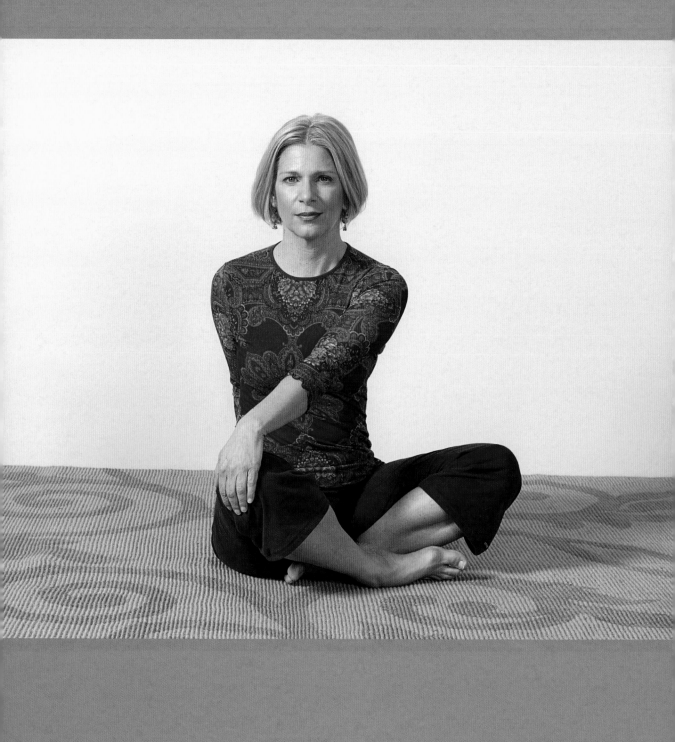

Foreword

Rita Trieger is one of those rare people (teachers) who can combine the Eastern philosophies of yoga and meditation with a very active Western lifestyle. Through her own personal experiences, she can always relate to her students and give them the kind of direction that fits into their busy lives. If she can do it, being an editor, a yoga teacher, and a woman with a family life, then those around her are inspired to try as well. And they do. She teaches students ranging from chronic overachievers to those who are chronically ill. She touches each life in a different way because she uses her deep understanding of yoga to lead her with each person.

Watching those who are in her classes return week after week religiously, gaining from her teachings, I can see improvement not just in their flexibility but in the way each person enjoys his or her life. Rita is a great teacher because she has a true belief in what she does, combined with a sense of humility.

She isn't forcing the body to conform, but allowing each participant to progress based on what he or she brings to his or her practice. Having worked with Rita for many years, I am glad that this book will be able to bring the joy of yoga, and relief from back pain, to so many more people. Her openness to learning is catching. So many who want to try yoga are inhibited by back pain and inflexibility. Through these simple daily programs, each person can gain the benefits I have seen in all those who are blessed to have her in their lives.

Elaine Petrone
Program Director
The Health and Fitness Institute, Tully Health Center, Stamford Health System
Author of The Miracle Ball Method, *Workman Publishing*

Introduction

One cold, lazy winter day, I wrapped myself in a blanket and settled into an afternoon of cable TV and hot tea. I felt tired but completely comfortable as I reached for the remote, when suddenly there was a hot flash of pain shooting through my left lower back. The pain was so sharp I felt as though I couldn't catch my breath, let alone move. After several minutes, I managed to gently rock myself up into a seated position but couldn't straighten up beyond halfway. I had to shuffle my way to the bathroom, bent over, to look for Ben-Gay. I felt like I was about 100 years old, and I couldn't stop whimpering. What was going on? This had never happened to me before. I was in good condition. I went to the gym six days a week, I was a personal trainer, I had never experienced any kind of injury before and certainly hadn't ever had the slightest twinge in any part of my back.

What I didn't know was that I wasn't alone. According to recent studies, more than 80 percent of the population will experience low back pain at some point in their lifetime. Many people end up having only a few episodes, while others develop lingering problems. Back pain doesn't discriminate; it affects men and women equally. Age isn't a factor either—it can occur at any age, striking most frequently between the ages of twenty-five and sixty. And because the human spine is so complex, the exact cause of acute low back pain is often easily masked. Pain can come from origins as varied as muscle trauma, nerve damage, infections, inflammatory diseases, and circulatory disorders, among others.

But for most of us who fall in the 80 percent zone, the best way to treat back strain and pain is to take a few days of rest and then get right back into action. It's also recommended that you start a plan of gentle exercise to stretch the muscles and keep the blood and oxygen flowing. It can be something basic like swimming or walking, or, better yet, a complete mind/body makeover with yoga.

Let's face it—life can be overwhelming. Most of us can't stop running long enough to take a significant break; clear the mind; and release some of the anxiety, frustration, stress, anger, and fear we deal with on a daily basis. When we don't deal with it, we end up storing stress in the body—pushing the tension aside until some later time, when, hopefully, we can sort it all out. More often than not, we end up burying it deep within our body's handy storage bins: the neck, shoulders, middle back, lower back, and hips. This stored tension in the body can result in weakness, exhaustion, illness, or chronic pain.

That's why yoga is such a useful tool for dealing with back problems. It teaches us to breathe more deeply, to consciously connect with the body and eventually release all the pent-up aggravation.

The simple 10-minute yoga practices in this book will help you to tune in to your body, let go of tension, relax tight muscles, and will even help relieve some developmental disorders such as scoliosis. However, if you have persistent, chronic, or severe back pain, it's always wise to check with your doctor before you start any sort of exercise program. The practices are gentle, but your doctor will be able to let you know if you need to avoid anything specific.

As for me, after about a week or so, my low back pain was gone. Thankfully I've never again had that kind of pain, although as I get older, I do find myself feeling soreness in the back from time to time—especially if I've been working at the computer all day or if I'm tired. When that happens, I get onto my mat and into one of my favorite yoga poses (down dog). Then I breathe deeply, let go of the negative thoughts that inevitably float through my brain, and let my body blossom into beautiful openness.

CHAPTER ONE

Anatomy of the Back

Think of your back as a powerhouse for
the entire body—it enables movement of your head, arms, and legs
and provides support for the trunk. And the human spinal column
is one of the most vital parts of the body—its excellent design serves
many bodily functions. For example, the spinal column and vertebrae
protect the spinal cord, which provides essential communication to the
brain, affecting the body's mobility and sensations through the interaction of the bones, ligaments, and muscles of the back and the nerves that
surround it. But keep in mind that the vertebrae and their joints can
each move in about six different directions, and all of that movement
means there's a fairly good chance that at some point, something is
bound to go wrong.

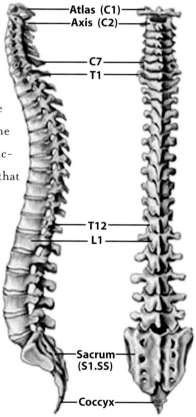

Atlas (C1)
Axis (C2)
C7
T1
T12
L1
Sacrum
(S1.SS)
Coccyx

The Infrastructure

We're born with thirty-three separate vertebrae, but by the time we reach adulthood, most of us only have twenty-four. That's because during normal development, vertebrae fuse together in certain parts of the spine. Each vertebra is shaped in a special way so that when they are stacked together, the spinal cord is protected by the bones of the entire spinal column.

The cervical spine is made up of the first seven vertebrae, C1 to C7, in the spine. It starts just below the skull and ends at the top of the thoracic spine. The cervical spine has a backward C shape and is much more mobile than either the thoracic or lumbar regions of the spine. Unlike the other regions of the spine, the cervical spine has special openings in each vertebrae for the arteries that carry blood to the brain.

The thoracic is the chest level region of the spine, which is located between the cervical and lumbar vertebrae. It consists of twelve vertebrae, T1 to T12, that serve as attachment points for ribs, and for this reason, it is the least movable part of the spine.

The lumbar spine, which holds most of the weight, consists of five vertebrae, L1 to L5, and it's in this area that most back problems happen. Right below the lumbar spine, the nine vertebrae at the base grow together. Five vertebrae form a triangular bone called the sacrum. Most people have two dimples in the low back, and this area—where the sacrum joins the hipbones—is called the sacroiliac joint. The lowest four vertebrae, which are fused, form the tailbone, or the coccyx.

Running through the center of the spine is the spinal canal, and through the canal is the spinal cord. The spinal cord is a collection of nerves that carry messages to and from the brain, relaying actions and sensations such as temperature, muscle control, and pain.

Common Back Ailments

Backache is one of the most common complaints among adults, and low back pain is the most prevalent cause of disability in people under the age of forty-five. The spinal region, from the neck to the buttocks, is especially susceptible to muscle, ligament, or bone injury. But with proper care—including maintaining correct posture and avoiding physical stress—acute or chronic backache can be avoided.

Although most back problems are musculoskeletal, kidney infections, gastrointestinal distress, reproductive organ problems, and other internal disorders can be the cause of some back pain. That's why it's so important to check with a doctor if you are experiencing prolonged or persistent pain.

Mechanical and Developmental Disorders

LOW BACK PAIN: Most often affects young adults or people in early middle age. Symptoms vary from morning stiffness to sudden side pain and the inability to stand up straight. Usually caused by strained ligaments and/or muscles or an intervertebral disk that has slipped. (Disks absorb the shock of motion.) Treatment for low back pain varies according to injury, but generally, maintaining good posture and regular exercise can help to greatly reduce low back problems.

LORDOSIS AND KYPHOSIS: Lordosis refers to the forward or inward curvature of the spine; usually affecting the lumbar (lower) region. Very common among obese people, lordosis can occur during pregnancy and can sometimes be caused by incorrect posture.

Kyphosis is an excessive curvature in the thoracic (upper middle) region, which can result in the condition usually referred to as hunchback. Kyphosis is very frequently associated with scoliosis, a lateral curvature of the spine. It can sometimes occur due to an injury to the back or by congenital malformation.

HERNIATED DISK: Pressure is exerted on the disk as the spine bends, which can cause the soft center (nucleus pulposus) to rupture through the outer ring (anulus fibrosus). This rupture then presses on a nerve running from the spinal cord to another part of the body. The pain is felt in the area that the nerve supplies. The area of the back most commonly affected is the lumbar region, because those disks take the most strain. If this occurs, the pain is felt in the buttock and down the leg to the foot, resulting in a condition called sciatica. Herniated disks are more common in young men than women.

COCCYGODYNIA: Persistent, severe pain in the lowest area of the spine, the coccyx. The pain increases during defecation and when sitting but reduces when the person stands. It can last for a few months and is generally caused by falling heavily backward and landing in a sitting position.

SCOLIOSIS: Some curvature in the neck, upper trunk, and lower trunk is normal—in fact, humans need the curves to help the upper body maintain proper balance and alignment over the pelvis. But side-to-side (lateral) curves are abnormal. Most often occurring in childhood, scoliosis is a curvature of the spine to one side. It can be caused by an alteration in the position of the underlying bones or by a reaction of the spinal muscles. Both can make the spine temporarily change position. If diagnosed early, measures can be taken to reduce severity. The most common form of scoliosis is adolescent idiopathic scoliosis (AIS), which develops in young adults around the onset of puberty. Scoliosis can also be the result of injury. Avoiding use of the injured area causes a person to compensate his or her posture, which can result in scoliosis.

SCIATICA: A pain that begins in the hip and buttock and continues all along the sciatic nerve, running into the back of the thigh and all the way down the leg, is referred to as sciatica. The condition is sometimes accompanied by low back pain, which can be more or less severe than the leg pain. Onset can sometimes be sudden and is usually caused by pressure on the sciatic nerve, which may be a result of a herniated disk or osteoarthritis.

If you have persistent back pain or you think you may have a specific back condition, please see your doctor immediately. Self-diagnosis or improper diagnosis may result in more serious injury.

Quick Reference Glossary

Here are a few terms that might be familiar but not quite clear to you:

ACUTE—Severe, for a short time.

BACK PAIN—Nonspecific term used to describe pain below the cervical spine.

CARTILAGE—The hard, thin layer of white glossy tissue that covers the end of bone at a joint. This tissue allows motion to take place with a minimal amount of friction.

CERVICAL—Of or relating to the neck.

CHRONIC—Frequent recurrence or long duration.

COCCYX—The small bone at the end of the spinal column in man, formed by the fusion of four vertebrae. The three, and sometimes four, segments of bone just below the sacrum; referred to as the tailbone.

DISC—Cushion of elastic tissue found between the vertebrae of the spinal column. These shock absorbers protect the spine from impact. Sometimes they can bulge beyond the vertebral body and compress the nearby nerve root, causing pain. The terms slipped disc, ruptured disc, and herniated disc are often used interchangeably even though there are subtle differences.

HERNIATION—Formation of a protrusion.

JOINT—The junction or articulation of two or more bones that permits varying degrees of motion between the bones.

LIGAMENT—A band of flexible, fibrous connective tissue that is attached at the end of a bone near a joint. The main functions of a ligament are to attach bones to one another, to provide stability of a joint, and to prevent or limit some joint motion.

LUMBAGO—A nonmedical term signifying pain in the lumbar region. Archaic term meaning back pain.

LUMBAR—The lower part of the spine between the thoracic region and the sacrum, the lumbar spine consists of five vertebrae. These five moveable spinal segments of the lower back are the largest of the spinal segments.

ORTHOPAEDICS (*also* ORTHOPEDICS)—The medical specialty involved in the preservation and restoration of function of the musculoskeletal system that includes treatment of spinal disorders and peripheral nerve lesions.

OSTEOARTHRITIS—Arthritis characterized by erosion of cartilage, which becomes soft, frayed, and thinned with bone and outgrowths of marginal osteophytes. To a certain degree this condition is unavoidable, but its onset can be delayed with exercise.

OSTEOPOROSIS—A disorder in which bone is abnormally brittle and less dense, and is the result of a loss of bone mineral as well as a number of different diseases and abnormalities.

SACRAL—Five fused segments of the lower spine, below the end of the spinal column, that connect to the pelvis.

SACRUM—The sacrum consists of five vertebrae that have fused together to form a single bone mass. The sacrum and pelvis (ilium) connect through the sacroiliac joints. The bottom of the spine, the coccygeal region, consists of four vertebrae that, like the sacrum, have all fused together to form the coccyx or tailbone.

SCAPULA—A large, triangular, flat bone lying over the back of the ribs on either side.

SPRAIN—An injury to a ligament that occurs when the joint is carried through a range of motion greater than normal, but without dislocation or fracture.

STRAIN—To injure by overuse or improper use.

TENDON—The fibrous band of tissue that connects muscle to bone. It is composed mainly of collagen.

CHAPTER TWO

Understanding Back Attacks

Remember the story

about my back attack? One back-breaking movement—reaching for a glass or bending to pick up a sock or, in my case, grabbing the remote control—is not the true culprit when it comes to pain, even though it may seem like it. That single occurrence is simply the straw that breaks the camel's back!

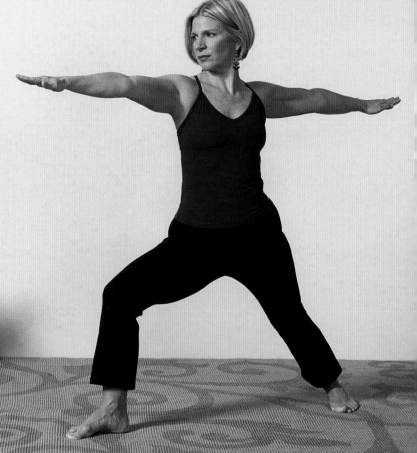

Keeping Muscles Healthy

The spine is surrounded by muscles, which give support, keep the spine stable, and enable it to move in different directions. It makes sense that in order to maintain a healthy spine, it's necessary to maintain healthy muscle balance where the spine and its nerves can be protected from stress and move freely without any hindrances. When muscles stop working correctly, problems are sure to occur. This can happen for many reasons, but most of the time it's due to incorrect body alignment or incorrect body positions that are held over a long period of time. This prolonged stretch causes muscle weakening, which then forces other muscles to take over.

For many of us, muscle imbalance is the cumulative effect of poor body awareness and bad posture. It could be that you just joined a gym or started a new activity, or that you continually do the same activity and use the same set of muscles over and over again. Ultimately we're all in the same boat; either we push our bodies too far, always overstraining or overreaching, or we don't push enough, never getting enough exercise and spending way too much time in the same sedentary positions. And let's not forget about stress. When we feel anxious or stressed, we tend to tense our muscles. This can cause headaches, tight shoulders, neck soreness, and even a tight jaw. If we never do anything to release this daily tension, it builds up and continually contributes to muscle imbalances.

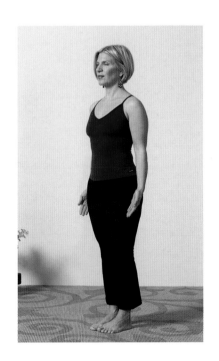

Posture Perfect

Wouldn't it be lovely if we could always stand with our weight evenly distributed through the body with all the joints resting perfectly in their neutral zones? It is attainable, I promise you. It just takes awareness and a little effort on your part.

Stand with the feet hips' width apart and make sure that the lower leg is vertical and at a right angle to your foot. Keep the knee joints in a line but don't lock them—keep them bent ever so slightly. Keep the pelvis neutral, with the hips over the knees, and let your spine curve naturally. Ribs are soft and breathing is easy and efficient. Keep the shoulders open by squeezing the shoulder blades together gently and then letting them drop down. Finally, keep your head neutral—not tilting too far back or too far forward, centered between the shoulders. Don't you feel better? You're probably even a little taller now!

Easing Pain

For more severe or
persistent pain:

- Apply an ice pack (or
  even a bag of frozen
  veggies will work) for
  a day or two to curb
  pain and swelling.
  Then switch to a
  heating pad (set on
  low) to promote blood
  flow, or you can use
  a deep-heating cream
  rub for temporary
  relief.

- Use an anti-
  inflammatory drug
  such as aspirin or
  ibuprofen to help
  relieve mild to
  moderate pain.

Pain Management

Pain occurs as a response to a signal sent to the brain. These signals are transmitted via the nerves, and they are a necessary warning that something is wrong. There are many ways that pain can manifest—it can be constant, recurring, dull, burning, or sharp. Depending on your problem, you may also feel a tingling or "pins and needles" feeling in your legs.

Pain is also classified as either acute or chronic. A sudden, sharp sensation is acute. It warns of imminent danger or bodily threat. Chronic pain is dull, warning us of disease or bad body function. Acute pain will usually block out chronic pain because the brain can't receive both messages at once, but the chronic pain will return once the acute has subsided. While acute back pain usually heals within a month or so, chronic pain is less responsive. The good news is that chronic low back pain can usually be managed with regular yoga practice.

Back pain can be mechanical or medical. Mechanical disorders of the spine are usually related to overuse such as poor posture or injury such as a herniated disk. These disorders are caused by local problems of the bones, joints, tendons, ligaments, muscles, and nerves of the low back. The position of the spine and activity of the person will affect the degree of pain. Most mechanical problems improve with time, and only a very small percentage of cases ever require surgery.

Sometimes pain from a back problem is referred, meaning that you may feel pain in one part of your body but the problem is somewhere else. If the problem is mechanical, the pain is usually felt in the center of the back or off to one side, with succeeding attacks occurring in the butt, the outside of the thigh, into the knee, and sometimes below the knee to the ankle or foot.

Common Culprits

Most back pain complaints originate in the low back. Low back pain can often be attributed to complex origins and symptoms, and can also begin in other regions of the body, eventually attacking the muscles or other structures in the lower back. Sometimes low back pain can even begin in the nerves or nervous system. Other origins for low back pain include trauma, infections, degenerative disorders, inflammatory diseases, circulatory disorders, or any of thirty additional causes.

It is often difficult for physicians to pinpoint the exact cause of a patient's low back pain because of the complex composition of the human spine. Bone, discs, muscles, ligaments, tendons, and various other tissues are arranged like a three-dimensional puzzle to make up the spine. The complex makeup can easily mask the exact cause of low back pain.

Back strain caused by muscle, ligament, or tendon injury is one of the most common causes of back pain. It's not unusual for ordinary occurrences—such as a sneeze or a cough or bending to pick up something—to cause strain, or strain can be due to lifting an object that's heavier than your muscles or ligaments can actually support. Whatever the case, the damaged back tissues send a signal through the nervous system, alerting all the muscles. The alert protects the injured muscle by producing a muscle spasm, which tightens all of the muscles in the intricate spinal network even though only one was actually injured (it's kind of like a charley horse in the back).

Sometimes spasms can be quite severe. The pain can be overwhelming and even cause immobility. Because the spasms naturally occur in order to slow motion and decrease irritation to the injured muscle, the best way to relieve the spasm is to keep moving. Slow movement will allow the muscle to continuously test how far it can stretch and as the irritation is gradually relieved, the muscle will return to its normal tension. Simple yoga stretches will go a long way to release back strain, and you can supplement with a heating pad and some aspirin if the pain is very bad.

Dealing with Discs

By the time you reach thirty, back discs, which are supposed to be spongy cushions, start to resemble pancakes. These changes to the discs can cause severe back pain, which varies with each individual. Exercise is the primary treatment for disc degeneration (think yoga!). Keep in mind that if you begin to limit the movement in your spine, stiffness and fatigue will undoubtedly set in. If your disc is herniated or "slipped" (that's when the gel-like center protrudes through the front, back, or sides), it can irritate the spinal nerves in the spinal canal. The body identifies the protrusion as foreign matter and inflammation sets in. Over time, activated enzymes will slowly dissolve the herniated portion but may also affect the nearby nerve. Once the nerve is inflamed, sciatica is generated in the leg.

Sciatica refers to pain that begins in the hip and buttock and continues all the way down the leg. This condition is often accompanied by low back pain, which can be more or less severe than the leg pain. Sciatica that's caused by a herniated disc usually leads to leg pain that worsens when sitting and improves while standing or lying flat. Before the disc actually herniates, there may be episodes of low back pain since the outer "tire" of the disc is being stretched, causing tension. When the disc eventually herniates, the low back pain is replaced with pain that shoots through the leg and foot.

The term *sciatica* indicates that the sciatic nerve, which travels from the lower back through the buttocks and into the leg, is the cause of the pain. True sciatica is a condition that occurs when a herniated lumbar disc compresses one of the roots of the sciatic nerve. This type of low back pain is less common than other conditions that produce back pain. For instance, sporting activities, recreational activities, and heavy labor can cause back and leg pain, which is commonly misdiagnosed as sciatica.

The most common symptom of true sciatica is pain in the back of the thigh, lower leg, or foot that very often results in much more discomfort than the lower back pain. It's important to note that true sciatica will produce radiating pain that reaches beyond the knee. Very often a person will have a history of lower back pain beginning a few days or weeks before the leg pain occurs, then the leg pain becomes worse than the back pain, and in some cases the back pain will completely disappear.

Other Common Problems

Systemic illnesses such as fibromyalgia make up about ten percent of back pain and they don't get better or worse with time or amount of activity. Keep in mind that many of the internal organs such as the kidneys and bladder as well as blood vessels and lymph nodes are nestled against the lower back. Diseases that affect these organs can cause back pain, and if you experience other symptoms such as fever, severe bone pain in the middle back, or pain that worsens when lying down or at night, make sure you see your doctor to determine if illness is the culprit.

General weakness, balance problems, or difficulty walking can be caused by several different cervical spine issues; for example, problems with gait and balance may be due to the spinal cord's being squeezed by bone spurs, as well as other degenerative changes in the cervical spine. This condition, called myelopathy, affects the entire spinal cord and can be difficult to detect because it usually develops gradually and also occurs at a time in life when people are beginning to slow down a bit anyway. Other symptoms of myelopathy relate to things that require a fair amount of coordination, like walking up and down stairs or fastening buttons.

Reducing Your Risk

When it comes to health, most of us don't take the time to practice prevention, and it's especially true when it comes to back problems. We'll just wait until something happens and then try to prevent a recurrence. But once you've already had a back attack, you're at greater risk of having another. The second attack happens because people forget the lessons from the first attack and quickly return to bad habits—lifting the wrong way, overstretching, or sitting too long.

But if you can take some simple steps and remember to practice good body mechanics, get enough rest, and exercise regularly, you can avoid back problems.

Reduce your risk or
prevent back problems by:

- reducing stress

- giving up smoking

- losing weight

- sleeping enough

- lifting correctly

- learning to stay
balanced

- never overreaching

- pushing, not pulling

Keeping physically fit, especially by strengthening weaker back muscles, will greatly lower your back pain risk. This is essential for people whose jobs require heavy lifting or physical labor. Abdominal exercises are also important for decreasing risk as they help to protect the back from overload. Although obesity is not necessarily a back pain risk factor, it can promote a sedentary lifestyle, which will prevent you from doing exercise. Aerobic exercise such as walking, cycling, or fitness classes will get your heart rate up and generate heat, helping to burn calories and improve circulation, muscle tone, and flexibility.

When it comes to your diet, it's best to eat as healthfully as you can. Make sure you get plenty of antioxidants into meals by consuming lots of fresh vegetables and fruits that are good sources of vitamins A, C, and E (the major antioxidants). Green and yellow fruits and veggies are a good source of beta-carotene, so get plenty of apricots, spinach, and carrots into your meals.

Having a well-balanced, vitamin-rich diet will ensure that your body will stay strong so that, if you do suffer from an injury, your body will be able to efficiently repair damaged cells, contributing to a faster recovery.

Practicing good body mechanics is as simple as standing up straight. Maintaining good posture will go a long way to balance and support the spine. When lifting an object, keep your feet and back facing the same direction (no twisting!). Always face the object, bend at the knees, and lift with your legs, not your back. If you lift a lot of heavy objects, you might want to invest in an abdominal corset. It'll give you a little extra support.

If you've ever had to stand for any great length of time, you may have noticed how tired the muscles in your back can become. This upright posture increases the curve in the lumbar spine and stretches the psoas muscle that travels along the front of the hip. To relieve the tension, transfer weight from foot to foot or flatten your back with a pelvic tilt.

If you find yourself sitting for long periods of time, make sure your seat height isn't too high. Your feet should be able to rest on the floor and your knees should be at an angle slightly above 90 degrees. If you have back pain, it's best to sit in a chair that has a firm, straight back and arm rests. Soft chairs or sofas will not give your back proper support, and you'll have to make too many adjustments, which will result in fatigue or even increase pain.

Overall you can avoid back pain by making an effort to never stay in one position for too long at a time. It doesn't matter if you're standing or sitting—just change the position once in a while. Constant muscle contraction causes fatigue, and if muscles are tired, they will ache. Aching muscles are weaker, and weaker muscles are at a greater risk for injury.

CHAPTER THREE

Understanding Yoga

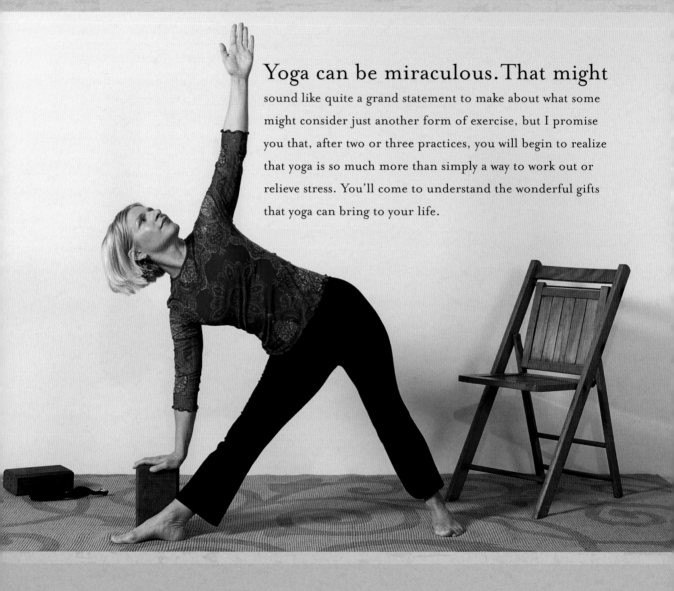

Yoga can be miraculous. That might sound like quite a grand statement to make about what some might consider just another form of exercise, but I promise you that, after two or three practices, you will begin to realize that yoga is so much more than simply a way to work out or relieve stress. You'll come to understand the wonderful gifts that yoga can bring to your life.

Start at the Beginning

The first and most important thing you need to do is open your mind and heart and make a commitment to your yoga practice. Remember that each person starts out with different needs but with the same apprehensions. A star athlete may have more overall ability but may not be able to let go of muscle tension and relax into a pose the way someone who has not been training for years can. Yoga levels the playing field and every person—from the weakest to the strongest—can walk away from his or her daily practice feeling restored. And you can spend as little as five or ten minutes a day practicing. As long as you do something, you'll begin the process of undoing years of damage.

The study of yoga is based on five thousand years of observations and theories involving the mind/body connection. When you practice regularly, the mind and body integrate, which enables you to heal both emotionally and physically as you create internal harmony. In time, you'll see that yoga not only helps to evenly distribute energy throughout the body, but also helps bring balance to the circulatory, respiratory, nervous, digestive, reproductive, and excretory systems.

How the Poses Do What They Do

Yoga poses deal with specific bodily needs and are able to direct blood and oxygen to the areas that are lacking, restoring healthy function and vitality. Conscious breathing refreshes the mind and removes dullness. As a result, when the body is balanced and our minds are clear, we become more positive, more confident, more peaceful, and more alive.

This may sound like clichéd mumbo jumbo, but the fact is that modern science and medicine are proving over and over again that making this important connection between mind and body is the key to effectively healing and balancing all the systems of the body as well as the mind. When the mind is overworked and overstressed, it fires off confusing and conflicting signals to the body, causing stress and imbalance. This imbalance in the body can cause weakness, exhaustion, or illness, which often results in the inability of the body to respond to the mind.

Your Own Personal Journey

It may be that your intention when you start a yoga practice may not include any thoughts about making connections or healing anything. You may simply be looking for a less jarring form of exercise—a kinder, gentler approach. If that's so, then yoga is truly the perfect choice. The movements in yoga bring stability and tranquility to the body as well as the senses. The brain and the body work together and energy is balanced throughout the body and mind. Yoga poses will stimulate but never irritate the body/mind. For example, a runner is able to increase his or her heartbeat, but the physical strength and endurance required can leave the runner exhausted as well as cause repetitive injuries to the joints and ligaments. In yoga practice, backbends are physically demanding; the heart is stimulated just as in running, but it beats at a steady, rhythmic pace, resulting in rejuvenation and renewed energy instead of fatigue.

The exertion in yoga is evenly distributed through all body parts, and because the body remains relaxed as you extend, bend, and stretch muscles and joints, it's protected from injury and stress. Postures also improve blood flow to every cell in the body, revitalizing and strengthening the nervous system and increasing the body's capacity to endure stress.

By using your own body weight, holding poses, and breathing rhythmically, you'll tone the whole body, strengthen bones and muscles, correct posture, improve breath capacity, and increase energy.

Eventually, though you may not be aware of it at first, your mind will become calmer and more focused, and an overall sense of well-being will begin to wash over your everyday life. You'll find that tasks become less difficult and obstacles are much easier to overcome. You'll be able to prioritize and let go of all those unnecessary negative thoughts and emotions. Think of yoga as a refreshing cleanse for the body, mind, and soul.

How Yoga Works

If you're used to the standard menu of gym classes, you might wonder how an environment that includes soft lights and soothing music could possibly help strengthen your body. And if you're not a regular exerciser, you might think that weary bones, stiff joints, and an overworked mind won't ever be able to relax, stretch, or perform what sometimes look like seemingly impossible poses. But remember that yoga's primary aim is to quiet the mind and restore the body. It's that simple. Those crazy, contorted poses that are often portrayed are only for the accomplished, been-practicing-for-years student. Keep in mind that no matter what level of training we begin with, we're all putting forth the same effort when we practice; we're just at different starting points. In other words, a person who is finally able to achieve a simple forward fold is experiencing the same euphoria as another person who is, at long last, able to gracefully lift into a handstand. Both people are able to accomplish specific or difficult individual goals, and in the process, both will discover a new understanding of their bodies.

How Yoga Soothes

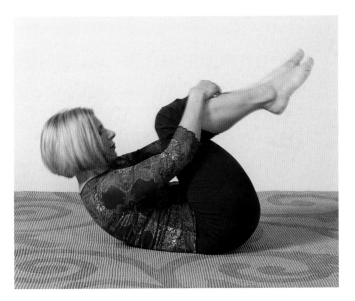

Reducing pain is often one of the main reasons why some people choose yoga. The poses, or asanas, work on specific body parts to soothe and restore but can also influence the chemical balance of the brain, improving your state of mind. For example, twisting poses such as Spinal Twist squeeze the internal organs, allowing fresh blood and oxygen to flush out toxins, while inverted poses such as Headstand or Shoulder Stand calm the body and stimulate the brain, and allow the heart muscle to rest and nerves to calm.

Because the back is made up of vertebrae and joints, each of which move in many different directions, the odds of something going wrong are much greater than with other body parts. Lower back strain is probably the most common back pain, and a big contributor is stress. It's not uncommon for a person suffering with undue stress to develop a muscle spasm just by bending to pick something up. In fact, many studies confirm that mental stress can and definitely does have an effect on muscles.

Simple yoga routines like the ones in this book will help to ease back discomfort and stress. Combining simple breathing techniques with these gentle postures will help get rid of knots, lengthen and release tight muscles, and melt worries away.

Breath Work

Breathing deeply and evenly is not only an essential tool for healing and releasing, it's the starting, middle, and ending points for every pose. The breath helps oxygenate every cell, strengthens the diaphragm, and eases pain; it can also fill you with energy or calm you down. By coordinating deep yogic breath with movement, you'll be able to stay focused and present in the moment—in other words, you'll become totally aware.

Always remember to keep the breath moving in and out through the nose (many yogis will tell you that the nose is for breathing and the mouth is for eating!). This will keep heat inside the body, warm the muscles, and keep the blood flowing. Generally, you should inhale when performing the part of the posture that opens the body and exhale when the body folds or closes.

Let the length of your breath determine how deeply you sink into a pose. In the beginning you may feel out of breath, so take it only as deeply as you can and then begin again. Eventually you'll be able to complete a full breath and a movement in perfect sync.

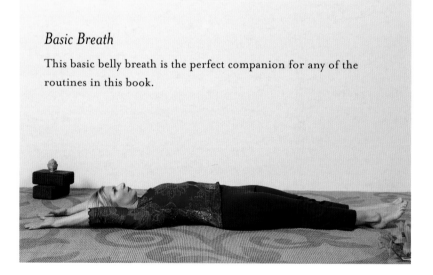

Basic Breath

This basic belly breath is the perfect companion for any of the routines in this book.

1. Begin by sitting or lying down comfortably. Place you arms at your sides, or if seated, rest them lightly on your knees. Close your eyes and begin to observe what's going on in your mind and body. Don't change anything about your breath—simply notice where it is and if it's getting stuck anywhere. Find your natural rhythm.

2. Slowly begin to lengthen each breath, matching the inhalations to the exhalations. Sometimes it helps to count. As you inhale, begin counting slowly to four or five, then exhale slowly to four or five.

3. Begin to expand the belly on each inhale, letting it fill completely like a balloon. On the exhale, draw the navel in (imagine there's a string tied to the navel that goes straight through your back, and now imagine someone pulling that string) and push every drop of breath out.

4. Continue breathing deeply for several more rounds. Notice that, with each breath you are able to soften and release specific tension points. Remember, wherever your focus is, your breath will naturally be drawn to that area. Use the breath as a tool to help warm and open up tight spots

Practicing at Home

Entering a class or yoga studio for the first time can be intimidating—especially if the other participants have been practicing for a while. So, it's completely understandable that, for many people just starting out, staying at home is the most appealing option. I agree it's a good idea (especially if it gets you to stick with it), but do plan on taking a class sometime soon. An instructor will be able to correct any misalignment and can answer any questions you may have about specific postures or problem areas.

For your at-home practice, you'll definitely need a sticky mat, and it might also be helpful to have a blanket, a block, and a strap handy in case you need some assistance or modification options.

A Sacred Space of Your Own

Before you do anything, find a room or a space in a room that can be rearranged easily for your practice. Perhaps there's a particular window where streams of morning sunlight or evening moonlight shine through. If you live in a city, windows may mean a lot of noise, so you might want to set aside an area that's tucked away and closed off. Whatever you decide, make sure you won't be disturbed and that you feel completely comfortable.

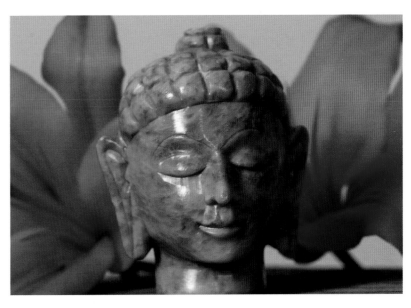

Set the tone of your sacred space by surrounding yourself with lovely things—maybe some flowers or a favorite object, or perhaps some scented candles. For example, I prefer evening practice and I love the beach and candlelight, so I always prepare an arrangement of seashells, whatever flowers are in season, and a few scented candles. I also like to include soft background music. You can pick popular artists or try some of the wonderful yoga and meditation music that's available. Most bookstores and music shops have a large selection.

Next, set aside a convenient time—if possible, the same time every day—to practice. Keeping to a regular schedule will help you to make a conscious commitment to your practice, even if it's only for five minutes. Most teachers and yoga masters agree that it's always better to do a little bit every day than to do two hours once in a while. With time and regular practice, you'll notice that your body will begin to crave yoga. And by taking the time to become familiar with the poses and the flow of your breath, tight spots will melt away, stored stress will be released, and any new tension will dissipate easily. Best of all, your body will begin to heal.

What to Wear

Very often, loose, comfortable clothing is recommended for practice, and that certainly is a fine option. However, I recommend you wear clothing that fits close to the body. I find pants and T-shirts that fit too loosely can get tangled, and you can't check on your alignment if you can't see where the cloth ends and your body begins! Of course, since some of the morning routines in this book can be performed in bed, pajamas are a fine option and will probably be the most comfortable way to practice.

Introduction to the Routines

All of the yoga postures in the routines that follow will help to stretch and strengthen your muscles and loosen tight joints. With regular practice you'll become stronger and more flexible, and you'll begin to release tension from stress-prone back and neck areas. Remember that for years our backs have had to sometimes carry the weight of the world, and it will take a bit of time to lighten the load and undo the knots. Give yourself the time, and you will be amazed at the long-lasting results: a limber, pain-free body.

Begin slowly and go into a pose only as far as feels comfortable for you. Keep your attention, focus on the breath, and don't let distractions into your mind. Every day of practice will take you farther into the poses, so be gentle and kind to your body.

Because weak stomach muscles can sometimes cause back pain, chapter 12 focuses on abdominal strength. Try to do these gentle yogic crunches every day or at least every other day to build up the abs and create a solid support system for the back

You can choose to do one or two routines a day—perhaps one in the morning and one at night—or you can do a different routine every day. As you become stronger, you can incorporate Sun Series (chapter 13) to create a more vigorous practice. If you start to feel really strong, you can create a longer practice by doing four or five of the routines in a row, since they are designed to flow into each other or to stand alone. Make the practice yours— you have choices. As you become more familiar with the poses, get creative and mix and match poses or routines. Yoga should be fun and relaxing and invigorating. Explore your body, connect with your mind, and learn to love your beautiful self!

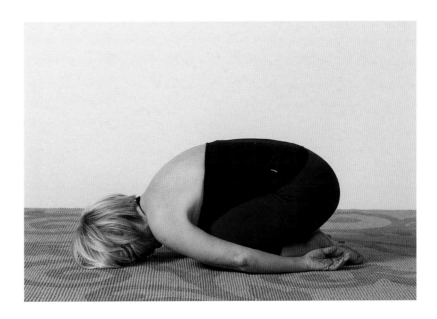

CHAPTER FOUR

Morning Stretch

Why not begin each day by being kind to your

body? Instead of jumping out of bed and rushing through your usual morning routine, give yourself a little love and comfort. You'll have plenty of time in your day to create stress! First thing: Shut off the alarm and take a moment to be thankful for another day. Then gently shift your focus onto your breath and take some deep inhalations and exhalations. Try not to think about what you need to do in your day and stay focused on breathing (don't fall back to sleep!). After a minute or two, begin to wake up the body with some yoga. You can perform these gentle morning stretches on your bed or on the floor—it's up to you. Just make sure you're comfortable. This sequence will take only five minutes, and you can surely spare this small amount of time to give yourself and your back a healthy start.

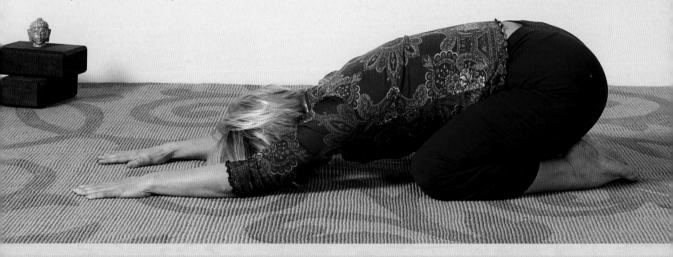

Reclined Mountain with Breath

The first part of your morning stretch is simple but requires your full attention. It's important not to let distractions interfere with your focus.

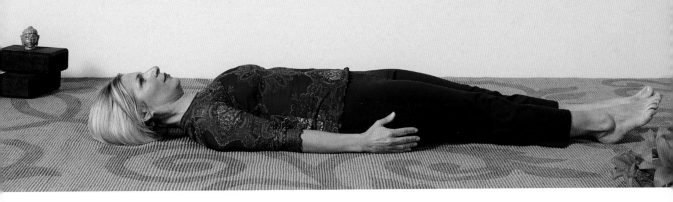

1. Lying on your back, squeeze shoulder blades together gently and draw them downward towards your butt, keeping your arms at your sides. Scoop your tailbone forward and try to rest the low back on the floor. Keep legs together, with feet flexed or pointed.

2. Breathe and observe. Notice if there is any soreness or tension in the back. Sometimes we sleep "wrong" and unintentionally strain muscles, so use your breath to awaken and let go of any tenseness.

Extended Mountain

You've probably done this stretch hundreds of times. But this time you'll be much more aware of what you're doing and of what's happening within your body.

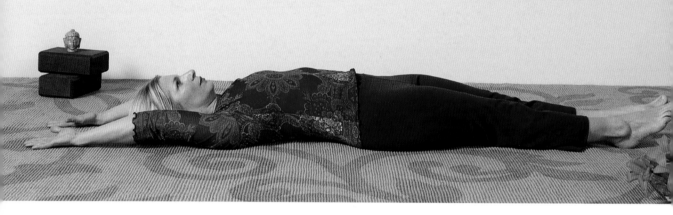

1. From Mountain Pose, extend your arms overhead, keeping shoulders down.

2. Extend outward through hands and feet, reaching in opposite directions and breathing deeply. Think about the legs moving out of the hip sockets and the arms moving out of the shoulder sockets. Every time you take another breath, reach a little further.

3. Add an extra stretch by alternating between the right and left sides and completely releasing in between.

4. Try to hold for five breaths during each movement.

Alternate Arm and Leg Raises

This flowing movement will begin to gently wake up the arms and legs and help to increase circulation.

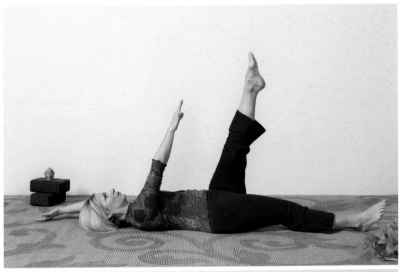

1. From Extended Mountain, exhale and slowly raise your right arm and left leg straight up to the ceiling. Feel yourself reaching upward through the toes and fingers and hold for three breaths.

2. Inhale and slowly lower, then raise your left arm and right leg, hold for three breaths, and lower.

3. Continue raising and lowering alternate arms and legs. Move as quickly or as slowly as feels comfortable for you, always moving with the breath. Try to complete five to ten repetitions on each side and rest back into Extended Mountain.

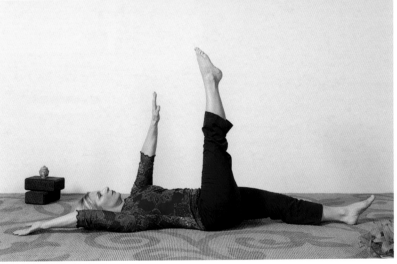

Gentle Bridge with Extended Arms

This version of bridge pose will awaken the spine and open up the belly. It also gently works the larger muscles of the lower body—the thighs, glutes, and hips.

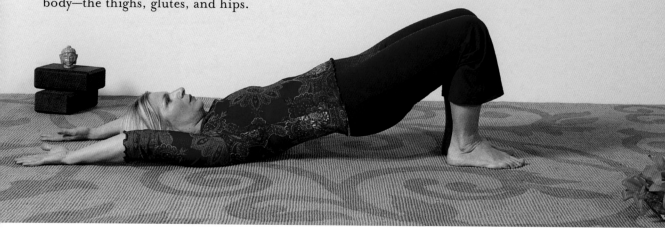

1. From Extended Mountain, bend your knees and place your feet flat on the floor at hips' width apart.

2. Scoop your tailbone forward and rest your low back as close to the floor as is comfortable. Pull your navel in, keeping your core center strong.

3. On an inhalation, press into the soles of your feet and lift your hips upward. Use your gluteal muscles to help lift.

4. Try to keep your hips and knees in line, not pushing the hips too far upward. Hold for two or three breaths, then draw the navel in and slowly lower, tucking the pelvis as you roll through each vertebra.

5. As soon as your tailbone touches the floor, press back into the feet and lift the hips again. Repeat this sequence three times. It should feel like a wonderful massage on the spine.

Supine Cat

Cat stretch is more often performed from a tabletop position, but this is a little easier on the back, making it a perfect morning stretch. This is a very subtle movement, so you'll need to remain very focused. It will stimulate and awaken the low back area, and it feels great.

1. After your last bridge, bring your arms down alongside your body, or if you prefer, keep them overhead.

2. On an inhalation, begin to gently press your tailbone into the floor as you gently arch the back.

3. As you exhale, draw the navel in and roll down through the low back as you scoop the pelvis.

4. Continue for as many repetitions as feel good to you.

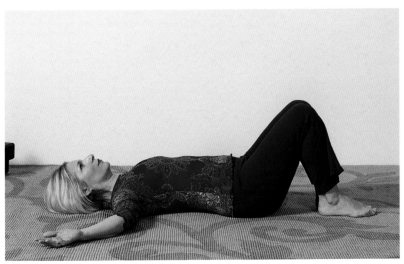

Hug Knees for Low Back Massage

A gentle movement to ease any low back aches.

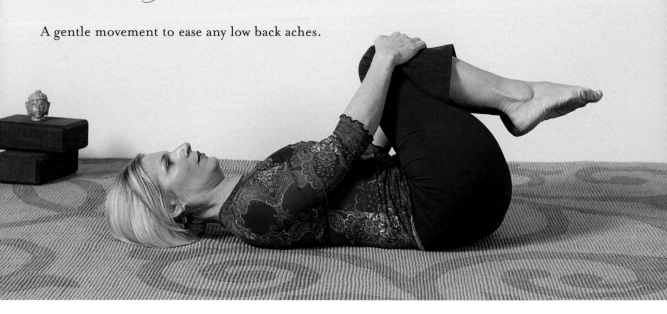

1. Hug your knees into your chest and hold for three breaths.

2. Place your hands on your knees and gently rotate your legs in a clockwise direction for as many rounds as you like, then come back to center.

3. Repeat the same movement in a counterclockwise direction.

4. Continue rotating and alternating as long as you like, and enjoy!

Lumbar Twist

This movement releases tension in the back. It feels really good any time of day, especially if you find yourself under unusual amounts of stress. Twisting in the morning will also help you let go of some toxins that might have pooled in the muscles while you were sleeping.

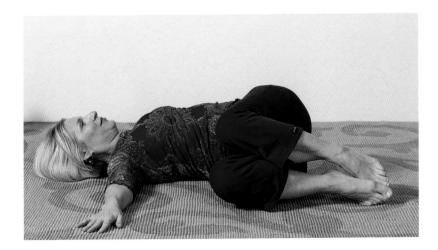

1. Hug both knees into the chest. Keep your legs tucked as you extend both arms out to either side of your body, with palms flat to the floor.

2. Lengthen your torso along the floor—reach the tailbone in one direction and tilt your chin toward your chest a bit as you extend outward through the crown of your head.

3. On an exhalation, drop both legs over to the right and keep both shoulders on the floor. Breathe. Feel the breath moving into the muscles of the back, bringing warmth and releasing tightness. Hold for three to five breaths, then come back to center and repeat to the other side.

4. When you've stretched both sides, you can continue to open up the back by continuing to drop the legs from right to left. Move slowly and always with the breath. When you've finished, roll to the right side and push yourself up to a seated position. Take another five breaths, then go ahead and begin your day!

The Morning Stretch Sequence

Move from posture to posture slowly and with your breath. If you find yourself feeling tense or beginning to worry about your day, relax into whatever posture you are in and take a few breaths before moving on to the next pose.

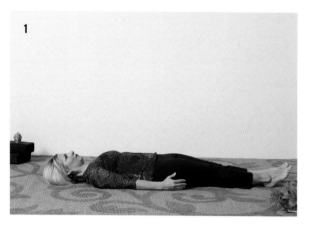

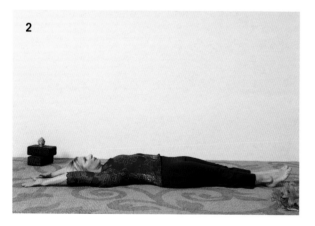

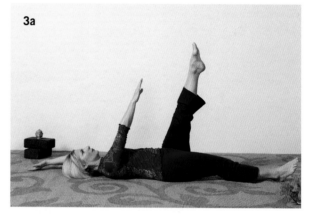

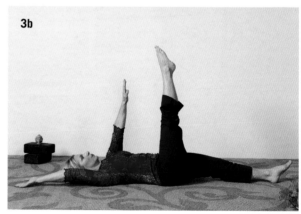

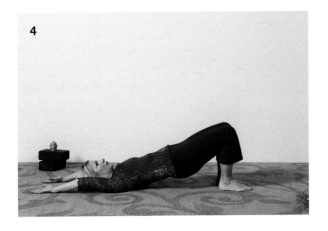

4

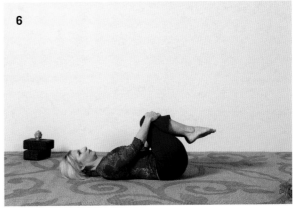

6

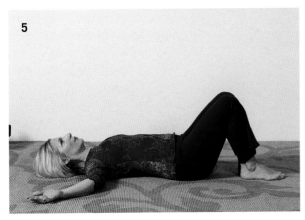

5

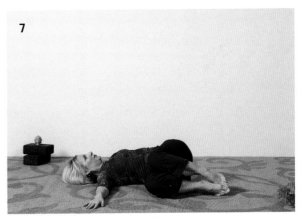

7

CHAPTER FIVE

Align the Spine

One of the most important

things you can do to avoid back problems and pain
is to maintain correct posture and spinal alignment.
This sequence will help to stretch and open up
constricted areas and allow your breath to soothe
and warm muscles, enabling them to release.

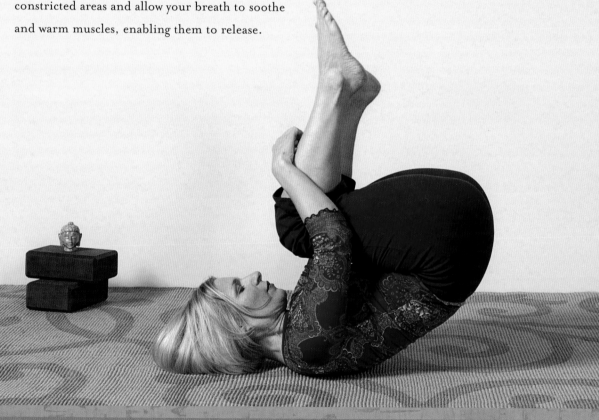

Reclined Mountain with Breath

This pose is simple but requires your full attention. It's important not to let distractions interfere with your focus.

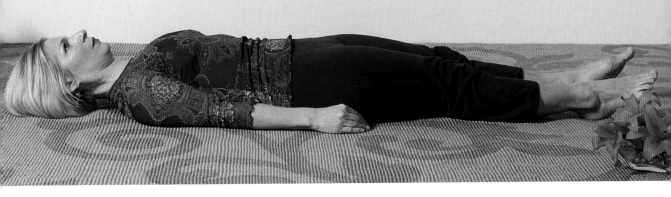

1. Lying on your back, gently squeeze shoulder blades together and draw them downward toward your butt, keeping your arms at your sides. Scoop your tailbone forward and try to rest your low back on the floor. Keep legs together, with feet flexed or pointed.

2. Breathe and observe. Notice if there is any soreness or tension in your back. Sometimes we sleep "wrong" and unintentionally strain muscles, so use your breath to awaken and let go of any tension.

Alternate Knee Hugs

This will release the low back. Take care to keep moving with your breath, always hugging on an exhalation.

1. Bend both knees and bring your feet flat to the floor. Make sure your back is resting comfortably on the floor, with a neutral spine—not too much of an arch and not too flat.

2. Bring your right knee in toward your chest and hold on to the front of your knee. Hold for two to three breaths and use the warmth of your breath to help open up tight spots.

3. Release on an inhale, then exhale and pull the left knee in. Continue to alternate for several rounds or until you begin to feel warmth and a gentle release in the low back.

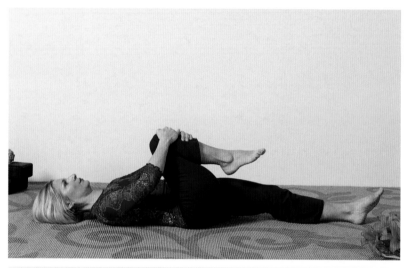

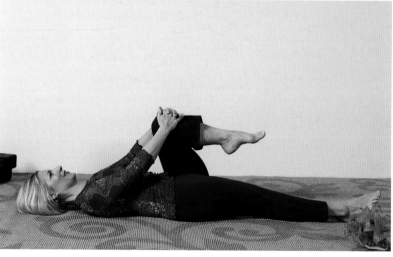

Spinal Twist

This should feel so good! It stretches the spine and shoulders; strengthens the low back; improves digestion; massages the internal organs; and relieves lower backaches, neck pain, and sciatica.

1. Hug the right leg into the chest with your hands holding onto the front of your knee.

2. Extend your left leg along the floor. Keep your head and neck aligned, and rest your spine in a neutral position.

3. Place the sole of your right foot gently onto the knee of the left leg.

4. Extend your right arm straight out from your shoulder with your palm flat to the floor, and place your left hand to the outside of your right knee.

5. On an exhalation, press your right knee over to the left and let your head roll right, setting your gaze over your extended arm.

6. Continue to breathe deeply and take the stretch as deeply as feels comfortable to you, always pressing further into the stretch as you exhale.

7. Return to center and switch legs, repeating the sequence on the other side.

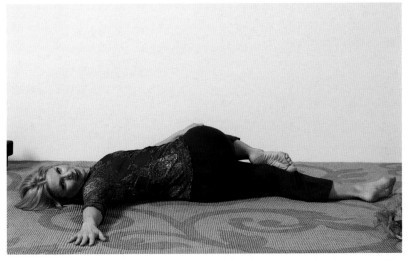

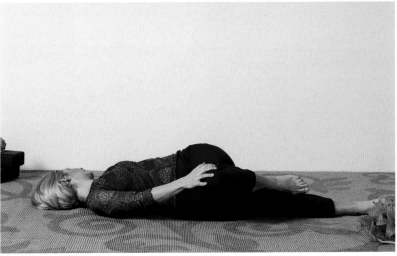

Happy Baby

Remember when you were little—before you had all the aches and pains—and you could have fun simply rolling around the living room carpet? I'm here to tell you that you can feel that joy again! Don't be surprised if you end up giggling, but keep in mind that you're also giving your kidneys a wonderful massage, you're stretching your hamstrings, and you're releasing the hips and easing back tension. Go ahead and enjoy.

1. Lying on your back, bring your knees in to your chest and place each hand on the front of each knee.

2. Open your knees all the way out to the sides, then, keeping your knees bent, let the soles of your feet face the ceiling.

3. Reach through your legs and hold on to your feet—one foot in each hand. If you prefer, you can wrap the first two fingers of each hand around the big toes.

4. Gently begin to roll from side to side. Push down on the feet, pressing knees toward the armpits, stretching the legs.

5. Continue rolling and stretching, letting yourself have fun as you nurture your body.

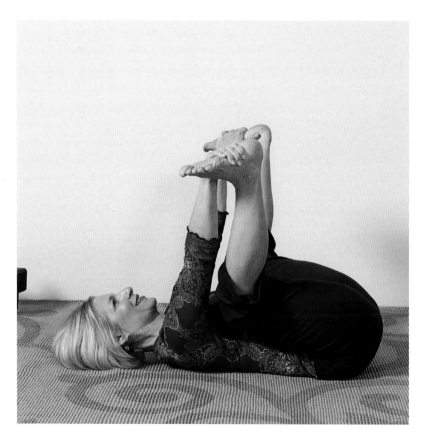

Cross-legged Roll-up

You'll feel like you've taken yourself on a ride as you gently rock back and forth. You'll be working your core center as you utilize abdominal muscles to initiate the rocking and rolling, plus you'll be getting a wonderful back massage. If you find that you can't get yourself upright this way, you can roll onto your right side and push yourself up to a seated position. Eventually you'll get strong enough to do the roll-up.

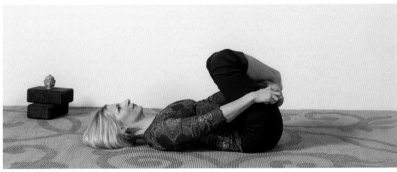

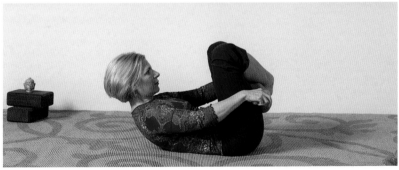

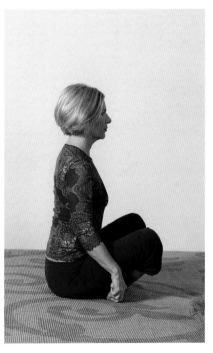

1. Lying on your back, hug both knees into your chest and cross your legs at the ankles.

2. Hold on to the big toes and begin to rock and roll back and forth.

3. Take the rocking and rolling into bigger and bigger movements until you can rock yourself right up into a seated position.

Simple Cross-legged Twist

A very simple move to begin to awaken and revive the spine. It reduces backache, neck pain, and sciatica. This will also help improve posture and digestion.

1. Sitting in a comfortable cross-legged position, pull the fleshy part of your butt away from your sitting bones. Feel the connection to the floor.

2. Place your hands on your knees and extend the spine as your reach out through the crown of your head.

3. Place your right hand behind the right hip and your left hand on your right knee.

4. On an inhale, activate both arms as you press into the right hand, lifting up and out of the waist. Exhale and press the left hand against the right knee as you twist your torso around, letting your gaze set over the right shoulder.

5. Continue to breathe and twist. Deepen the twist on the inhales and release into the stretch on the exhales. Hold for three to five breaths, then come back to center and repeat to the other side.

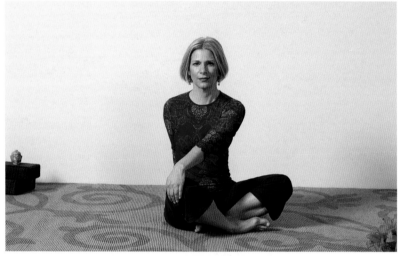

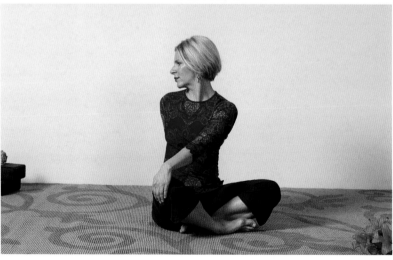

Seated Spinal Twist with Bent Legs

Seated twists will not only increase your energy level, but will also tone the internal organs, improving digestive and lymphatic systems. It will also alleviate sciatica and relieve backache, especially in the lumbar spine.

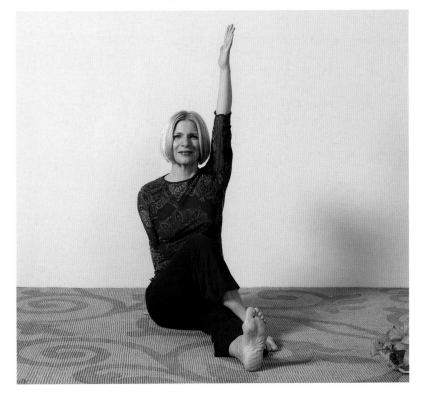

1. Come into a seated position with your legs extended straight out in front.

2. Move the fleshy part of your butt away from your sitting bones and feel the connection to the floor.

3. Bend your right leg and place your foot flat on the floor. Wrap your arms around your bent leg, using it as leverage to straighten your spine.

4. Find yourself reaching out through the crown of your head, with one long line of energy extending from your sitting bones up through your spinal column and out through the crown.

5. Pick up your right foot and place it on the floor to the outside of the left knee.

continued on next page >

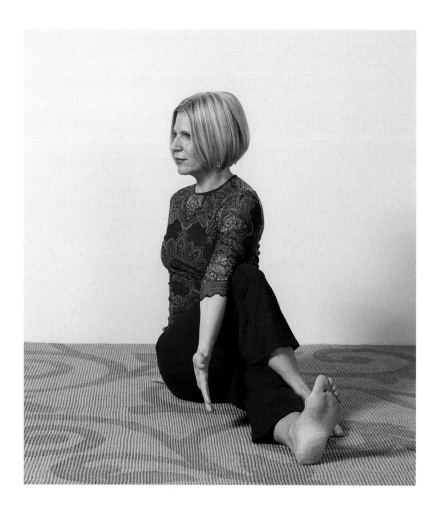

6. Place your right hand on the floor behind your right hip. Extend your left arm straight up, reaching out through each fingertip.

7. Inhale and extend your fingers further, lifting your ribs up out of the waistline.

8. Exhale and twist halfway to the right. Bring your left arm down and place it against the outside of your right thigh.

9. Activate both arms, and on another exhalation, press into your right hand as you press against your right leg and you twist all the way around, letting your gaze look beyond your right shoulder.

10. Don't stop twisting! Continue taking the pose deeper with each breath, lifting on the inhales and twisting on the exhales. Even if it's just a millimeter at a time, feel yourself squeezing your torso like a sponge. Wring out all the toxins.

11. Hold for three to five breaths, then slowly come back to center. Extend both legs and shake them out before repeating to the other side.

Transition: Rock and Roll to Floor

A fun way to get to the floor.

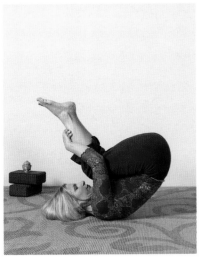

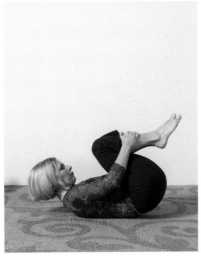

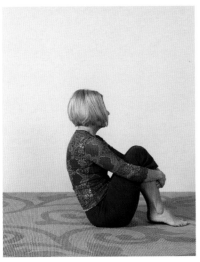

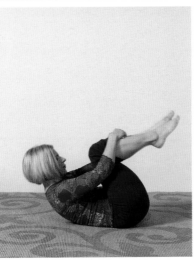

1. From a seated position, hug both knees into your chest and wrap your arms around them.

2. Begin to bounce off of the soles of your feet, letting each bounce roll you back and then forth. Let the bounce get bigger and the rocks will get bigger until you are rocking and rolling vigorously.

3. Rock and roll for as long as you like, then come to rest on the floor with your knees hugged in to your chest.

4. Turn your knees clockwise and then counterclockwise for a low back massage.

Sacral Twist (feet on the floor)

Another great tension reliever. It feels really good any time of day.

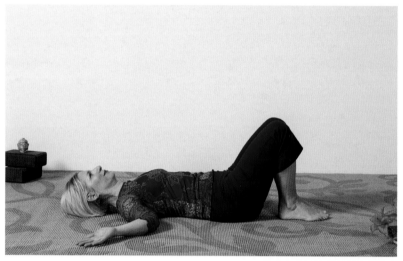

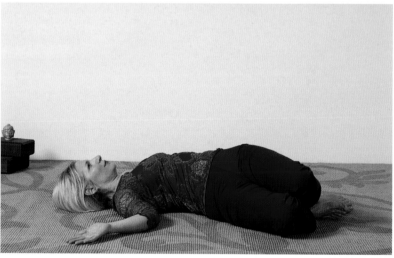

1. Bend both knees and keep feet together and firmly planted on the floor. Extend your arms out from your shoulders and let them rest on the floor, palms up.

2. Lengthen your torso along the floor—reach the tailbone in one direction and tilt your chin toward your chest a bit as you extend outward through the crown of your head.

3. On an exhalation, drop both legs over to the right and keep both shoulders on the floor. Hold for three to five breaths, then come back to center and repeat to the other side.

4. Continue to "windshield wipe" the legs from right to left, moving as quickly or as slowly as feels good to you. Enjoy the movement and your breath moving through the muscles.

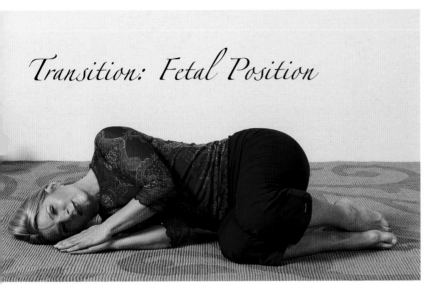

Transition: Fetal Position

From your back to your belly.

1. Roll onto your right side and let your head rest on the floor, hands in prayer position, with your knees tucked up and into your chest.

2. Rest here for a moment, and savor the nurturing feeling.

3. Roll over onto the belly and go right into Child's Pose.

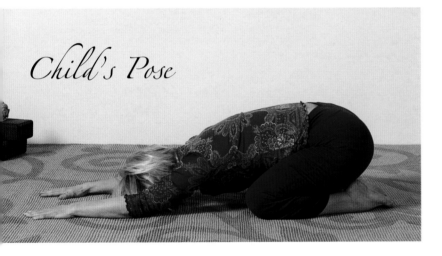

Child's Pose

1. From Fetal Position, extend your arms and fingertips along the floor.

2. Slowly walk your fingertips forward until your butt lifts up off the floor and you can pull yourself onto all fours.

3. Bring your big toes together and keep your knees wide apart.

4. Slide your hips back and let them rest on your heels, then extend your arms forward and let your forehead rest on the floor.

5. Relax and breathe.

This is such a nurturing, healing pose. It alleviates head, neck, and chest pain; opens the pelvic floor as well as the upper and lower back and hips; and reduces stress. Use it anytime you need a break from the chaos. Breathe into all the muscles and joints and surrender to the pose. Don't allow distractions or thoughts in. This is your chance to assess the body. Child's Pose is an inversion, so it will calm the central nervous system and help rest the brain.

Align the Spine Sequence

This routine gets you moving a little bit and you'll probably feel the difference in your back even after doing it just one time. I recommend doing it a few times in a row so that your heart rate goes up a little. This is a great way to get ten minutes of exercise into your day without having to head to the gym or for a walk around the block. Plus, of course, your back will feel great afterwards!

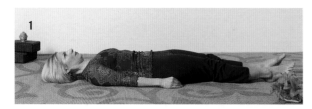

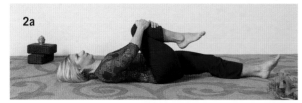

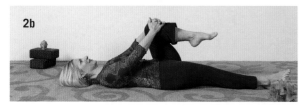

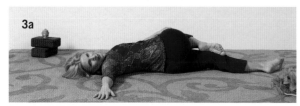

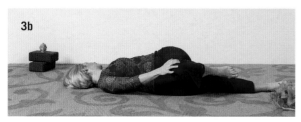

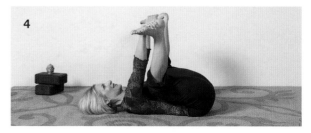

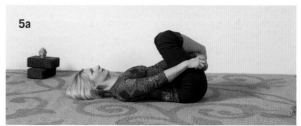

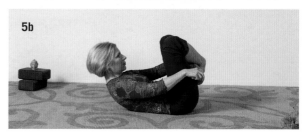

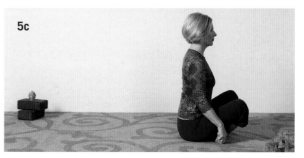

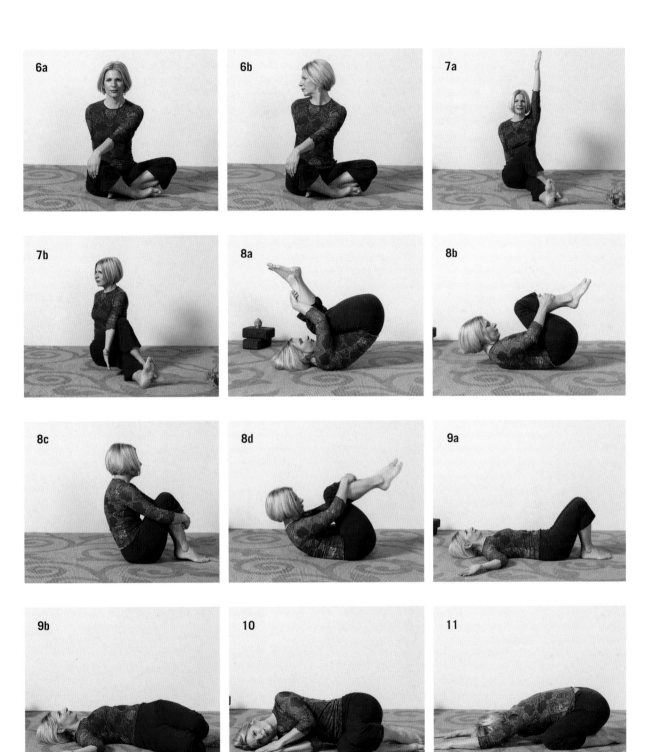

CHAPTER SIX

Backbends

Backbends stimulate the adrenal gland,

creating an abundance of energy throughout the body. They are completely
rejuvenating and will awaken the upper back, chest, shoulders, and groin
as they increase flexibility. They also present a wonderful opportunity
to release stress, and can do wonders for your posture. The muscles of
the back and spine are strengthened and digestion and circulation are
improved. Always remember to keep your breath flowing during backbends,
and never practice right before sleep, as they will energize your body.
Cool down and balance the body with forward folds.

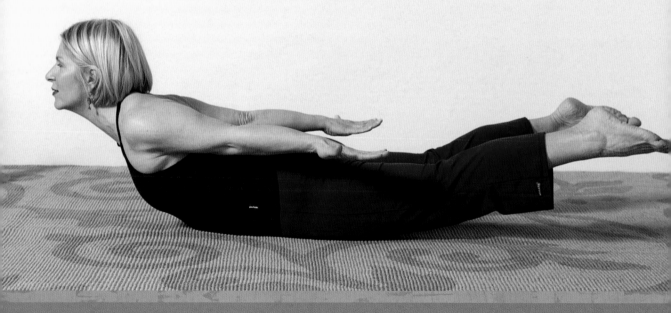

Child's Pose

Use Child's Pose anytime you need a break from the chaos or as a resting pose. In this sequence, feel free to go back to Child's Pose between each backbend. This will help to release any tension from the backbends and will also bring balance to your spine. Breathe into all the muscles and joints and surrender to the pose. Don't allow distractions or thoughts. This is a gentle movement to ease any low back aches.

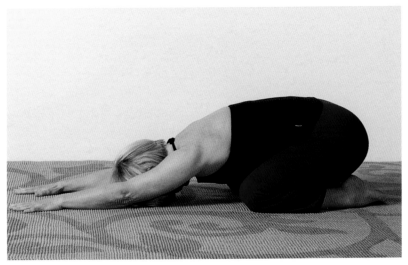

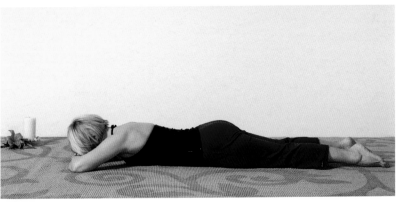

1. Bring yourself onto all fours; then bring your feet together, letting the big toes touch, and keep your knees wide apart.

2. Slide your hips back and rest them on your heels, then extend your arms forward and let your forehead rest on the floor.

3. Relax and breathe.

4. Look forward and slide body into prone Sivasana.

5. Release the weight of your body into the floor. You can rest your forehand on top of stacked hands or turn to one cheek with your arms resting at your sides. Hold for twenty breaths.

Sphinx

A gentle version of Cobra, practicing Sphinx will strengthen your lower back and help you sit up taller.

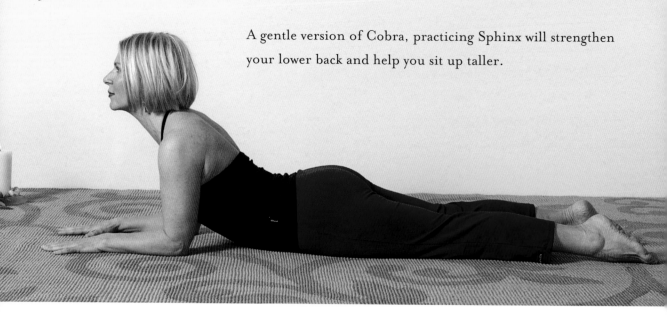

1. Lying on your belly, slide your hands underneath your shoulders. Keep your legs open to hips' width apart, with the tops of your feet resting on the floor.

2. On an inhale, press into your hands and slowly raise your forehead, nose, chin, and chest.

3. Make sure your elbows are under your shoulders. Spread your fingers wide. Breathe and hold the pose for three to five breaths.

Half Cobra

If you're not ready or strong enough to try Cobra, begin more gently in this modified version. You will reap all the same benefits—strong back, hips, and legs; improved posture; and energized mind and reduced stress—without the added stress.

1. Lie on your belly and bring your forehead to the floor. Bend your elbows and place your hands underneath your shoulders.

2. Keep the shoulder blades together and moving down toward your butt. Elbows should remain close to your sides and pointing up. Legs are hips' width apart, with the tops of your feet pressed to the floor.

3. Inhale and press the pelvis and legs down as you raise your head and lift gently through the heart center.

4. Look forward and feel the muscles of your back engaging. Keep the breath slow and even. Hold for three to five breaths, then release.

Cobra

Besides improving your posture, Cobra will strengthen your back, hips, and legs; stimulate the circulatory, digestive, and lymphatic systems; energize the mind; and reduce stress!

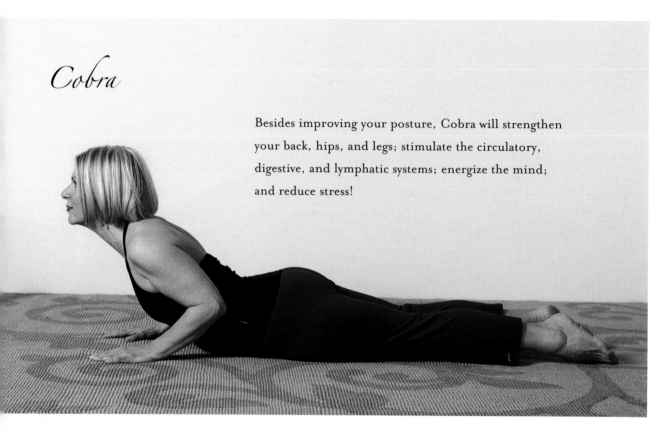

1. Lie on your belly and bring your forehead to the floor. Bend your elbows and place your hands alongside your body near the lower ribs.

2. Exhale and press downward into your palms as you lengthen your spine, and then squeeze the shoulder blades together, drawing them down toward your butt.

3. Press onto the tops of your feet and press your tailbone down. Inhale, and as you press your hands down, lift your torso up.

4. Keep your neck long, curling it to look upward. Hold for three to five breaths.

Modified Locust

Locust will help to energize the mind as it lengthens the spine and strengthens the legs, buttocks, shoulders, and arms. It increases flexibility, tones the abdominal wall, helps digestion, and improves posture.

1. Lie on your belly, with your forehead resting on the floor. Bend your elbows and place your palms alongside your body, at the low waist, just above your hip line.

2. Keep your feet about hips' width apart, and keep your shoulder blades drawn together and sliding downward toward your butt.

3. Inhale and lift your head, chest, and legs up off the floor as you press your pelvis and palms into the floor.

4. Breathe and hold for three to five breaths, then slowly release.

Flying Locust

Helps to energize the mind; lengthen the spine; and strengthen the legs, buttocks, shoulders, and arms. Flying Locust will also increase flexibility, tone the abdominal wall, help digestion, and improve posture.

1. Lie on your belly, with your forehead resting on the floor. Place your arms alongside your body, with your palms facing the floor.

2. Keep your feet about hips' width apart, and keep your shoulder blades drawn together and sliding downward toward your butt. Bring your arms away from the body slightly so that they form "wings."

3. Inhale and lift your head, chest, arms, and legs up off the floor as you press your pelvis into the floor.

4. Breathe and hold for three to five breaths, then slowly release.

Transition

Bring your hands under your shoulders, then push up and back into Child's Pose.

Child's Pose/Folded

This will alleviate head, neck, and chest pain; open the pelvic floor as well as the upper and lower back and hips; and reduce stress.

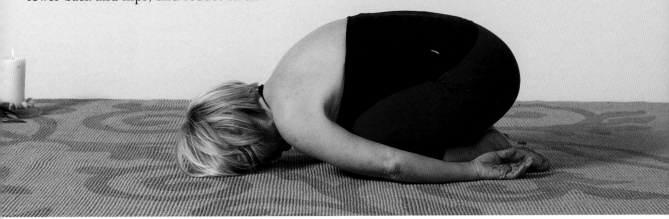

1. Bring the big toes together and keep your knees together.

2. Slide your hips back and rest them on your heels, then gently lower the torso and rest your forehead on the floor with your arms folded alongside your body.

3. Relax and breathe.

Rabbit

Considered an inversion, Rabbit or Hare pose opens up the entire back, neck, and shoulders. It is an excellent counterpose to more challenging backbending, and it will also improve circulation, calm the nerves, and improve your complexion.

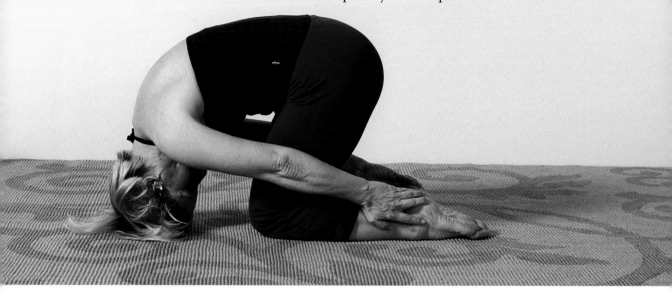

1. Slide your head closer to your knees, letting your forehead rest on the floor. Grab hold of your heels with your hands.

2. Pull yourself into a compact pod shape, making sure your forehead is as close to your knees as possible.

3. On an inhale, lift your butt and round through your spine as you roll onto the crown of your head. Breathe into your back and neck and use the warmth of the breath to soften muscles.

4. Hold for two to five breaths, then slowly come back down. Repeat two or three more times.

Transition

From Child's Pose, come to sit on heels, then shift hips to one side and swing legs forward.

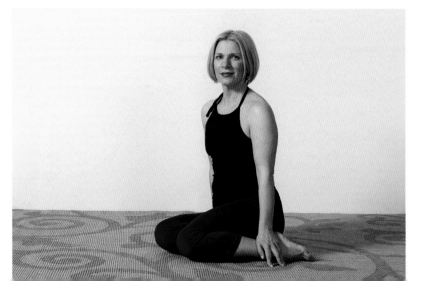

Seated Forward Fold

A counterpose to backbends, Forward Fold rests and massages the heart, soothes the adrenal glands, tones the internal organs, activates a sluggish liver, and improves digestion. It also stretches the spine, hamstrings, and calves; calms the nervous system; and alleviates high blood pressure.

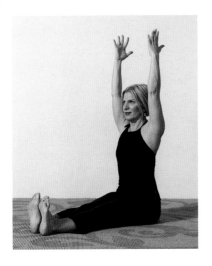

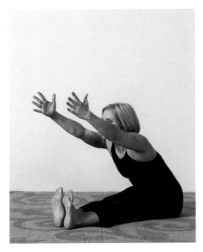

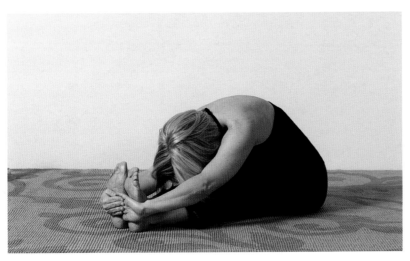

1. Sit with your legs extended along the floor, straight out in front of you. Move the fleshy part of your butt away from your sitting bones and feel the connection to the floor.

2. Extend your arms overhead, releasing any holdings in your shoulders. Reach through all ten fingers, sending energy upward.

3. Inhale and reach further, lifting the rib cage off the waistline.

4. Exhale and hinge at the hips as you fall forward. Keep your spine long and continue to extend through the fingers all the way down.

5. When you can no longer hinge, round down and release your arms, letting them rest on some part of your legs. Some people will be able to hold on to their feet while others may only reach their knees or shins. Know that wherever you are is exactly where you should be.

6. Breathe and let go of tension as you surrender to the breath and to gravity. Hold for three to ten breaths, then slowly walk yourself back up.

Backbend Sequence

Backbends are, to many yoga newcomers, the toughest poses to do and the most intimidating, and that's a shame, because if you sit at a desk all day or drive in a car a lot, you will probably eventually develop a forward bend in your back which can really wreck your posture. Therefore, backbends are highly beneficial to anyone who sits a lot and the variations in this chapter aren't very strenuous. This is a great series to do after work or after a long car ride.

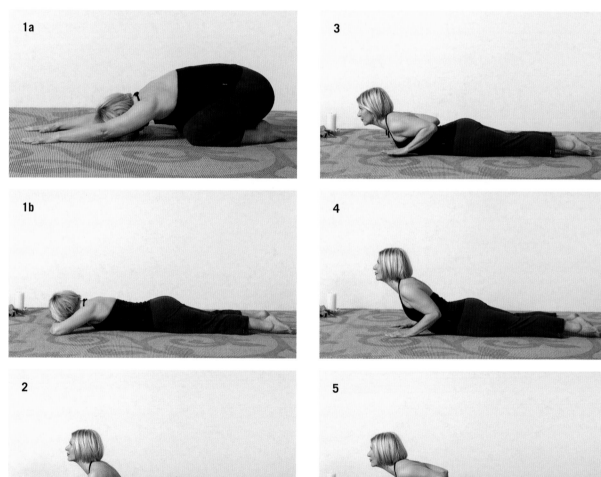

6

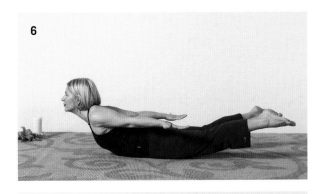

7

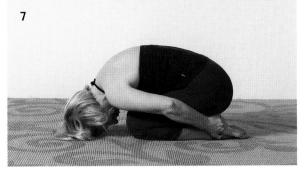

8a

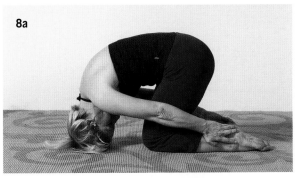

8b

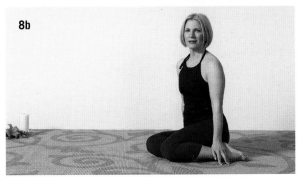

9a

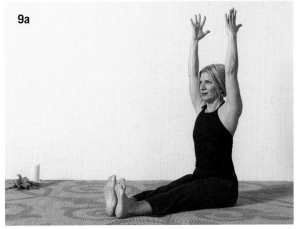

9b

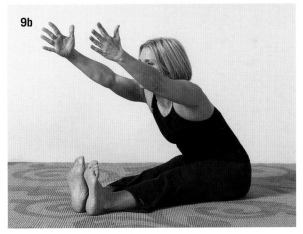

9c

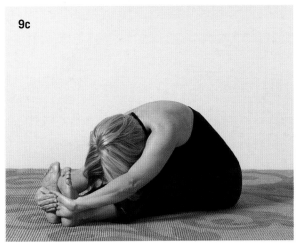

CHAPTER SEVEN

More Backbends

These poses are a little more challenging.

You can feel free to mix and match them with the simpler poses in the last
chapter, or you can leave some out and then add in more difficult poses
every time you practice or whenever you feel you are ready for more work.
Backbends create an abundance of energy throughout the body. They also
relieve stress, do wonders for your posture, tone the muscles of the back
and spine, and improve digestion and circulation. Always remember to
keep your breath flowing, as there is a tendency to hold the breath. It's
important to focus on continuing to move the oxygen and blood through
the muscles.

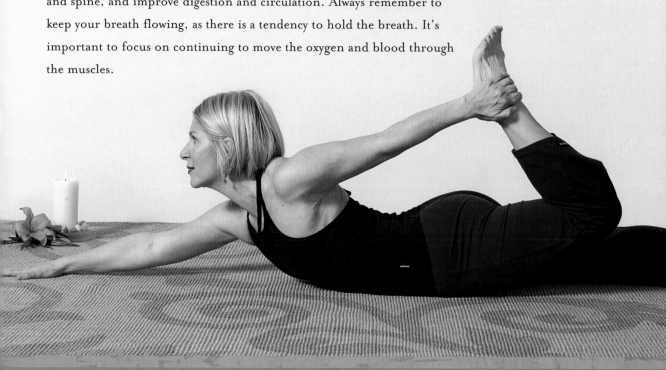

Gentle Bridge

This version of Bridge will awaken the spine and open up the belly. It also gently works the larger muscles of the lower body—the thighs, glutes, and hips.

1. From Extended Mountain, bend your knees and place your feet flat on the floor at hips' width apart.

2. Scoop your tailbone forward and rest your low back as close to the floor as is comfortable. Pull your navel in, keeping your core center strong.

3. On an inhalation, press into the soles of your feet and lift your hips upward. Use your gluteal muscles to help lift.

4. Try to keep your hips and knees in line, not pushing your hips too far upward. Hold for two or three breaths, then draw your navel in and slowly lower, tucking your pelvis as you roll through each vertebra.

5. As soon as your tailbone touches the floor, press back into your feet and lift your hips again. Repeat this sequence three times. It should feel like a wonderful massage on your spine.

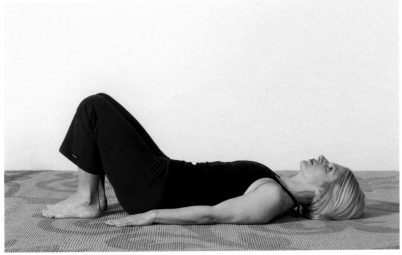

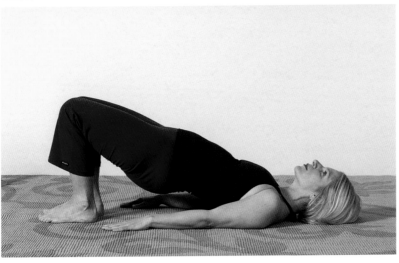

Full Bridge

Bridge will improve flexibility in the spine and shoulders and open up the chest and neck as it increases lung capacity. It will also help stimulate the central nervous system, the thyroid, and the parathyroid glands; relieve high blood pressure, asthma, and sinusitis; help with digestion; and reduce fatigue. You can see why this is a good pose to practice every day!

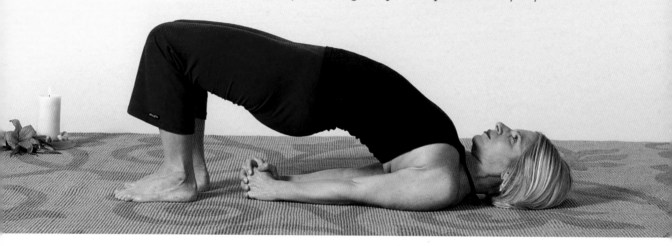

1. Lie on your back and place both feet on the floor, keeping them parallel and hips' width apart.

2. Keep your spine neutral, creating a natural curve. Inhale and press into the soles of your feet as you lift your hips up. Feel yourself lengthening through the tailbone and extending through your pelvis, straight through your knees.

3. Use the powerful lower-body muscles—your glutes, quadriceps, and hamstrings—to propel the hips higher, then roll the shoulder blades together and bring both arms underneath your body, interlacing your fingers.

4. Continue to press into your feet and keep your knees parallel (think about pressing a block between the knees—this is the correct knee position). Hold for three to five breaths.

5. Unclasp your hands and bring them to your sides. Slowly draw your navel in and curl your pelvis as you roll down very slowly. Take your time and feel each vertebra as you roll down, giving yourself a gentle massage.

Bridge with Crossed Leg

This Bridge variation allows you to increase the stretch in your hips and legs, while releasing your abdominal muscles.

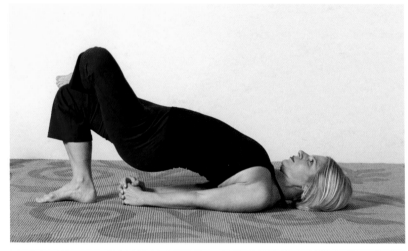

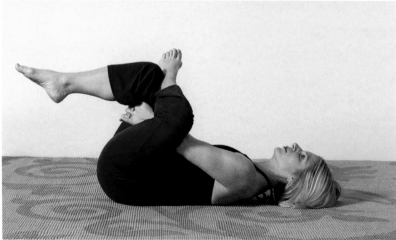

1. Lie on your back and place both feet on the floor, keeping them parallel and hips' width apart.

2. Cross your left ankle over your right thigh, making sure that your ankle bone clears your thigh.

3. Inhale and press into the sole of your right foot as you lift your hips up. Engage your right hamstring and gluteal muscle to lift you higher.

4. You can roll your shoulder blades together and bring both arms underneath your body, interlacing your fingers, or simply keep your arms at your sides.

5. Hold for three to five breaths; then slowly come rolling down through the vertebrae. As soon as your tailbone touches the floor, lift up your left foot, then grab hold of your right thigh and exhale as you pull your legs toward your face. Press your left elbow into your left thigh for a deeper stretch. Hold for three to five breaths and feel your right hip and left hamstring opening and lengthening.

6. Gently release, lowering legs to the floor; then uncross and repeat to the other side.

Rest: Reclined Bound Angle

(Supta Badha Konasana)

This restful pose is a great way to recharge between backbends. It will improve digestion and circulation; keep the prostate, kidneys, and urinary tract healthy; prevent varicose veins; keep the reproductive organs healthy; and relieve anxiety.

1. Lie on your back with bent knees.

2. Let the knees fall open and bring the soles of the feet together.

3. Scoop your tailbone forward and let your low back rest closer to the floor.

4. Relax into the pose and let yourself go. Feel the weight of your body, and with every exhalation, let go of anything that's no longer necessary in your life.

Modified Bow

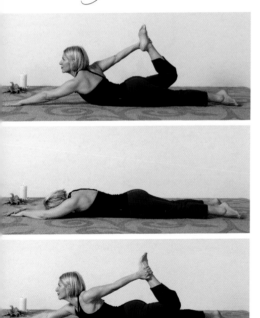

We're modifying Bow pose for this sequence, but you will reap all of the benefits from this intense backbend. Your whole body will be energized as you strengthen the spine, open the chest and throat, stretch the thighs, reduce stress, and relieve mild depression.

1. Lie on your belly with forehead to the mat, and extend your arms overhead.

2. Bend your right knee then reach around with your right hand and grab hold of your foot or ankle. (Your left hand remains overhead and your left leg remains extended.)

3. Inhale and press your pelvis into the floor as you press your right thigh up and back.

4. Look straight ahead and feel your right shoulder opening and stretching from the force of your foot pressing into your right hand. Feel the low back awaken as you hold for three to five breaths, then release.

5. Rest for three breaths; then repeat on your left side.

Camel

We hold a lot of the day's stress in our bellies, and this is a great way to open up the solar plexus and release anxiety. Camel will also stretch the thighs, torso, chest, shoulders, and throat, and strengthen the legs, pelvis, and lower back. It will stimulate circulation, improve posture and spinal flexibility, and energize the body and the mind.

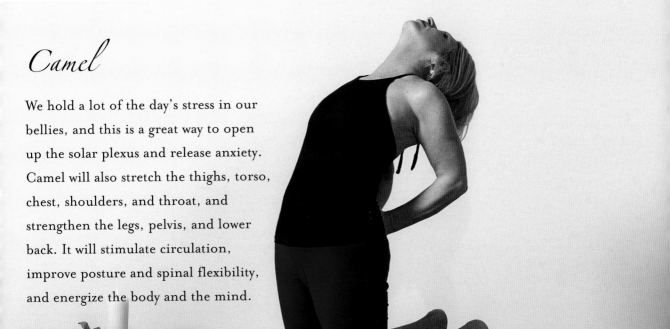

1. Kneel on the floor with your thighs parallel. Stack your hips over your knees and your shoulders over your hips. Scoop your tailbone down toward the floor to lengthen your spine.

2. Bring your shoulder blades together and slide them down your back. Place your hands on your low back (sacrum) with the fingers pointing up. If this feels uncomfortable, make fists and press the fists into your low back. Bring your elbows close together.

3. Inhale and press your hips and thighs forward as you press hands firmly into your back. Let the head drop back comfortably and breathe deeply.*

4. Hold for three to five breaths, then slowly come back to the start, supporting your back with your hands at all times.

*For more of a challenge, let your hands drop down and grasp your heels of your feet. Keep pressing forward with your hips and thighs and let the belly open up completely. Breathe deeply and hold for three to five breaths, then come up slowly, placing your hands on your low back and continuing all the way up to starting.

Child's Pose

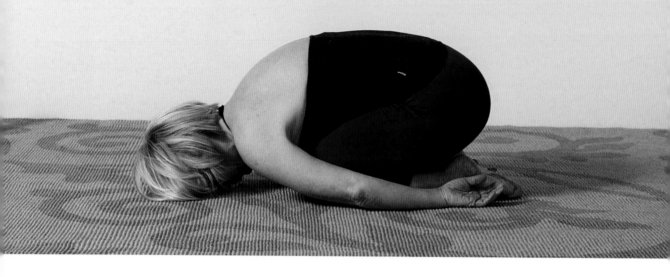

This is such a nurturing, healing pose. It alleviates head, neck, and chest pain; opens the pelvic floor as well as the upper and lower back and hips; and reduces stress. Use it anytime you need a break from the chaos. Breathe into all your muscles and joints and surrender to the pose. Don't allow distractions or thoughts in. This is your chance to assess your body. Child's Pose is an inversion, so it will calm the central nervous system and help rest the brain.

1. Bring yourself onto all fours, then bring your feet together, letting the big toes touch, and keep your knees wide apart.

2. Slide your hips back and let them rest on your heels. Extend your arms forward or alongside your body and let your forehead rest on the floor.

3. Relax and breathe.

Forward Angle

Forward Angle stretches the lower back, inner thighs, and hamstrings, while relaxing the upper back and front torso.

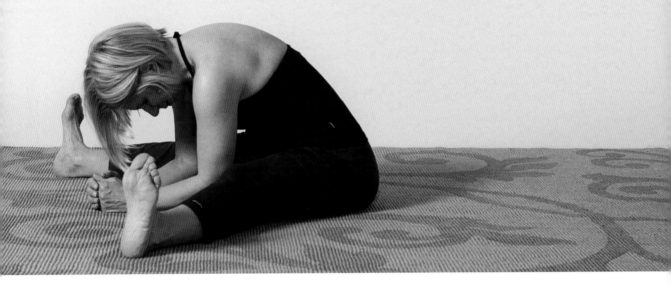

1. Sit with your legs extended along the floor, straight out in front of you. Move the fleshy part of your butt away from your sitting bones and feel the connection to the floor.

2. Open your legs and widen them out to your sides just until you feel a stretch in your inner thighs.

3. Put your hands and elbows on the floor and drop your upper body forward, releasing any tightness in the shoulders.

4. Exhale and hinge at your hips as you fall forward. Keep your spine long and continue to extend through your fingers, all the way down.

5. When you can no longer hinge, round down and release your arms, letting them rest on some part of your legs. Some people will be able to hold on to their feet, while others may reach only their knees or shins. Know that wherever you are is exactly where you should be.

6. Breathe and let go of tension as you surrender to the breath and to gravity. Hold for three to ten breaths, then slowly walk yourself back up.

More Backbends Sequence

These postures will truly begin to reverse any stooping or slumping you do throughout the day. But, more than that, backbends are known to open the heart, often stimulating a sense of openness for the yogi who practices them. When doing these postures, focus on releasing your front body (shoulders, chest, and torso) and allowing it to relax into the muscles of your back (which are doing the strengthening work). Many people begin to feel a sense of ease and relaxation in these postures which in turn relaxes their backs!

1a

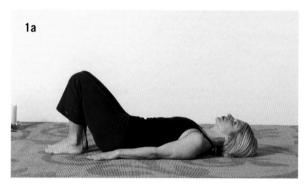

2

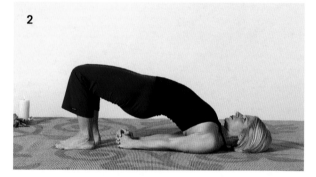

1b

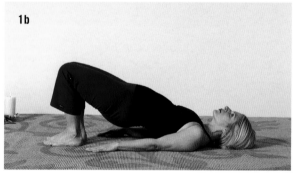

3a

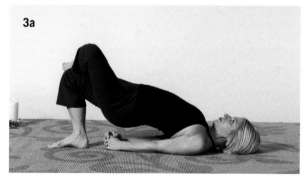

3b

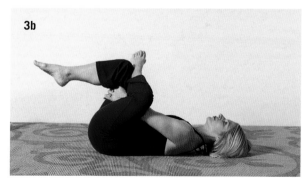

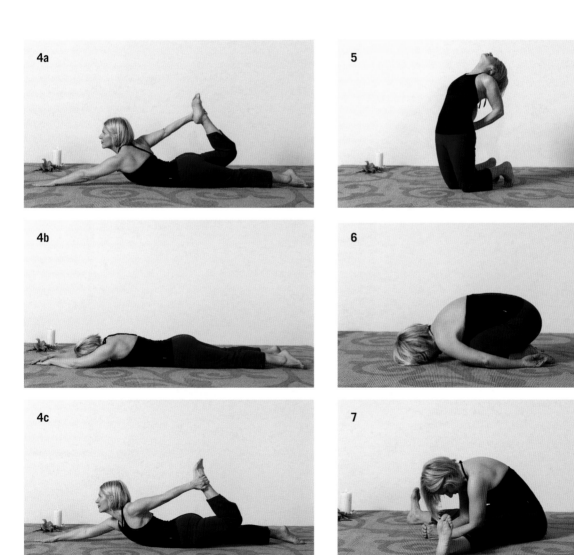

4a

5

4b

6

4c

7

CHAPTER EIGHT

Moving Forward

Forward folds soothe the central nervous

system and open up the entire back side of the body. They can relieve tension and improve digestion and elimination because they massage the internal organs and cleanse the liver and the intestines. If you do only one pose each day, make it a forward fold—it's that healthy.

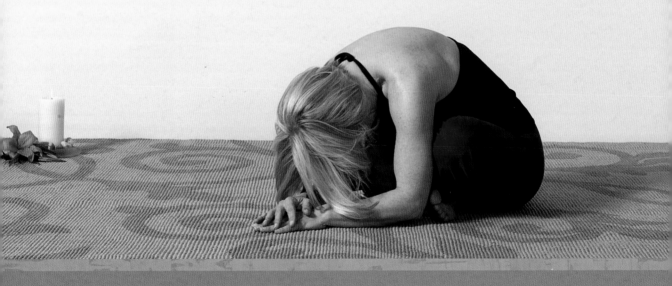

Child's Pose

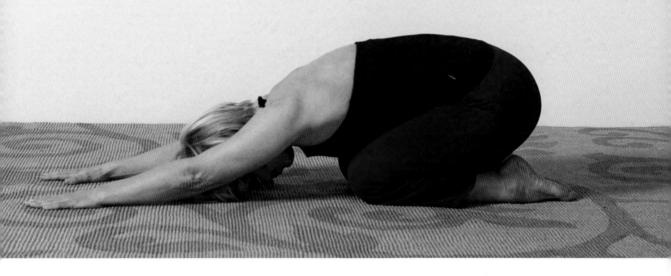

This is such a nurturing, healing pose. It alleviates head, neck, and chest pain; opens the pelvic floor as well as the upper and lower back and hips; and reduces stress. Breathe into all your muscles and joints and surrender to the pose. Don't allow distractions or thoughts in. Child's Pose is an inversion, so it will calm the central nervous system and help rest the brain.

1. Bring yourself onto all fours, then bring your feet together, letting your big toes touch, and keep your knees wide apart.

2. Slide your hips back and let them rest on your heels, then extend your arms forward and let your forehead rest on the floor.

3. Relax and breathe.

Down Dog

In a vigorous yoga practice, Down Dog plays an essential role as a transitional stage between poses. On its own, it will stretch the palms, chest, back, hamstrings, calves, and feet; strengthen the arms, legs, and torso; and energize the entire body. It can also improve focus and willpower, stimulate the mind, reduce stress, and relieve low back pain.

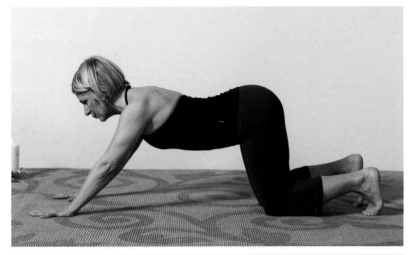

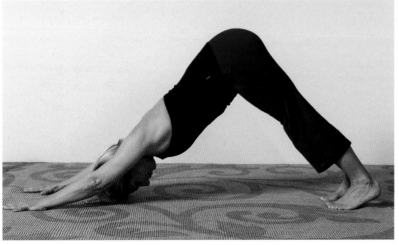

1. From Child's Pose, come up onto all fours. Walk your knees back slightly behind your hips. Place your hands directly under your shoulders and spread your fingers wide, with your middle finger pointing forward.

2. Press down into the roots of your fingers and think about drawing the shoulder blades together, then sliding them down your back.

3. On an inhalation, lift your hips and lengthen through your spine as you roll your shoulders open.

4. Keep a slight bend in your knees and scoop your tailbone even further up, then exhale and straighten your legs, sending your heels toward the floor.

5. Continue to deepen into the pose with every breath, making adjustments and letting your body begin to blossom open.

6. Hold for three to ten breaths, then drop back onto your knees and back to Child's Pose if you need a rest.

Standing Forward Fold

Strengthen the feet, knees, and thighs; stretch the hamstrings and calves; improve digestion; open up the hips and groin; and soothe the nervous system while you flush the brain with fresh blood and oxygen. All of these wonderful, healthy benefits by simply turning yourself upside down!

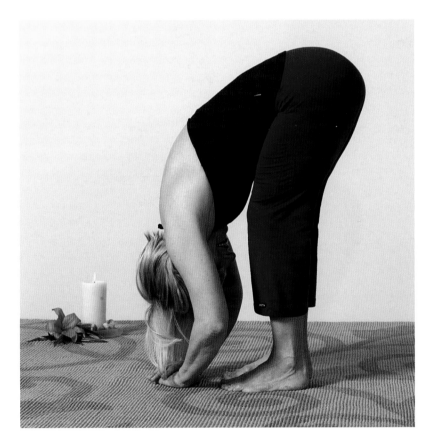

1. From Down Dog, bend both knees and walk the feet forward, keeping a bend in your knees to protect the low back.

2. Bring your awareness into the hinges of your hips, and think about elongating your torso and draping it over your legs. Release the crown of your head toward the floor.

3. Bend your knees deeply and rest your belly on your thighs. This will free the spine and allow you to release the weight of the upper body. Feel yourself surrendering completely.

4. Breathe deeply, letting go of tension with every exhalation. Shake your head yes and then no to release tension in the cervical spine.

5. Try to stay in forward fold for five to ten breaths, continuing to breathe deeply and release.

Chest Expansion

To open up the chest and stretch the muscles of the shoulders and arms.

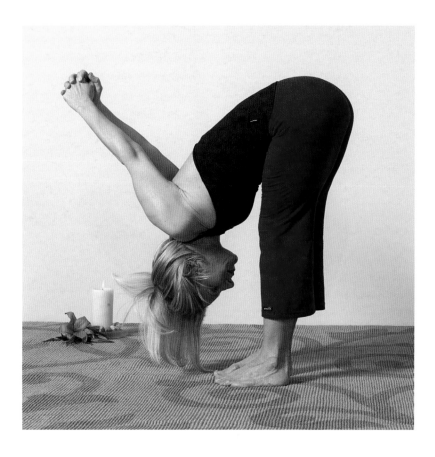

1. Sweep your arms behind your back and interlace your fingers. Extend your tailbone up to the ceiling, and let your arms fall overhead, surrendering to gravity and your breath.

2. Exhale and extend your tailbone up to ceiling, letting your arms fall overhead, surrendering to gravity and your breath.

3. Hold for three to five breaths, then pull your navel in and extend out through the crown of your head. Keep a flat back and let your arms pull you back up.

Hindi Squat

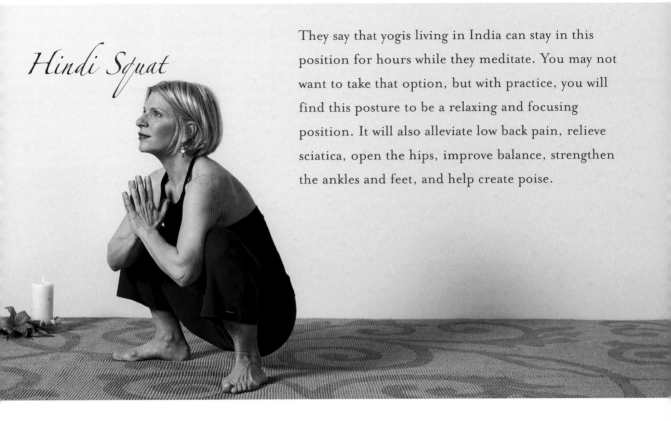

They say that yogis living in India can stay in this position for hours while they meditate. You may not want to take that option, but with practice, you will find this posture to be a relaxing and focusing position. It will also alleviate low back pain, relieve sciatica, open the hips, improve balance, strengthen the ankles and feet, and help create poise.

1. From Forward Fold, let your hands rest on the floor between your feet, and heel-toe the feet open to wider than hips' width.

2. Bend knees deeply and drop the tailbone down. Brace your arms against the insides of your knees and bring your hands into prayer or namaste position.

3. Breathe and release into the pose. Let your tailbone continue to drop, and keep pressing your arms against your legs, opening them further as you sink deeper.

4. Close your eyes and relax for five to ten breaths, or longer if you prefer.

Transition

Fall back onto your butt and bring your legs into comfortable cross-legged position.

Seated Forward Fold with Crossed Legs

Be very careful not to force this move. If you're especially tight or tense, this may feel uncomfortable at first, so always listen to your body. Use your breath and gravity to help you ease into the pose. Give yourself time and remember that with every practice you'll melt deeper into it.

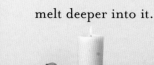

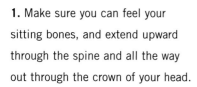

1. Make sure you can feel your sitting bones, and extend upward through the spine and all the way out through the crown of your head.

2. Keep your shoulders directly over your hips, then extend your arms overhead, reaching through all ten fingertips. Make sure your shoulders drop down, away from your ears.

3. Inhale and feel your rib cage lifting up off the waistline.

4. Exhale and hinge at the hip joints, continuing to extend through your fingertips as you slowly fold forward.

5. Go as far as you can, keeping your spine long, then round down and let your hands rest on the floor. If possible, bend your elbows and let your forearms rest on the floor.

6. Let go of tension in the head and neck, and soften the shoulders and the middle back. Continue to breathe slow, even breaths, relaxing deeper with each exhalation.

7. If your arms are long and extended, you can gently walk your fingers forward on an exhalation and work the pose deeper.

8. Continue to relax and breathe for five to ten breaths, then slowly come back up or go into the next pose.

Head-to-Knee Pose

Open up the chest and lungs; improve your digestion; increase your circulation to the liver, kidneys, and colon; alleviate headaches; and strengthen your low back. You'll also relieve stress, anxiety, and mild depression.

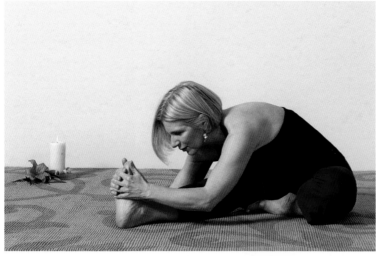

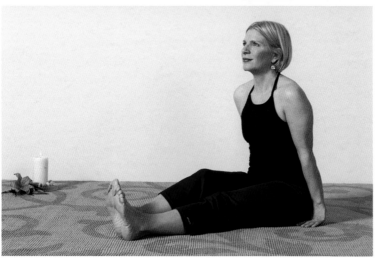

1. From a cross-legged position, extend your right leg straight along the floor and press the sole of your left foot up against your right inner thigh. (If this feels uncomfortable, you can rest your foot lower on your right leg.)

2. Turn your torso to face your right leg and extend your arms forward. If you can reach your foot, then hold on to it. If you're not quite there yet, hold onto your leg wherever feels comfortable. You should be challenging yourself but not forcing the stretch.

3. Inhale and lengthen up through your spine; then exhale and extend your torso forward, leading with your heart center.

4. If you are able, let your forehead rest on your shin. You can also modify the stretch by bending the knee of your extended leg and letting your belly rest on your thigh.

5. Breathe and release any holdings or tension with every exhalation. Feel yourself completely let go.

6. Hold for three to ten breaths. Then slowly come back up and repeat to the other side.

Transition
Bring legs together and shake out.

Moving Forward Sequence

What could be more relaxing than rolling forward into a ball? For many
yogis, Child's Pose, and other forward bends are the most restful postures of
all. To make these poses work for you, remember that forward bends allow
the back to stretch, releasing tense muscles. While relaxing into all postures
is a wonderful thing, you will also want to focus on feeling your body use the
poses in a purposeful manner.

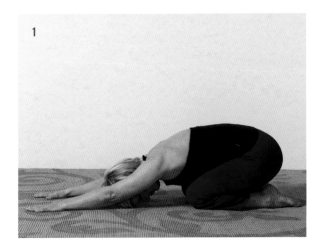

1

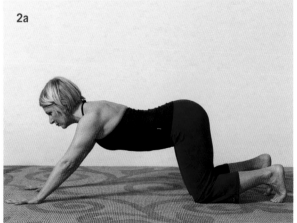

2a

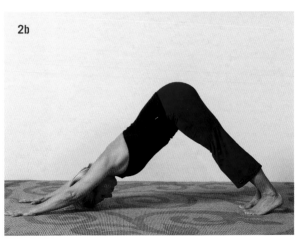

2b

3

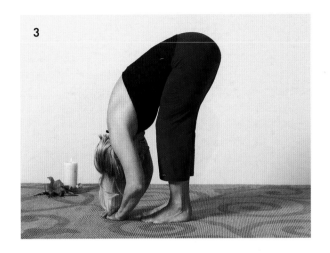

6

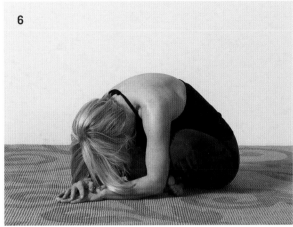

4

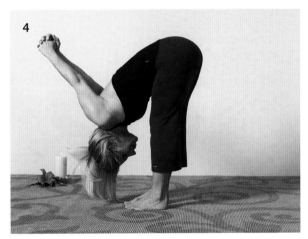

7a

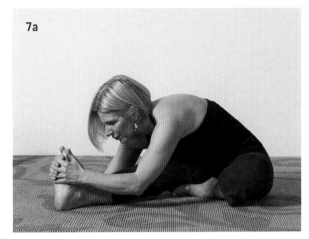

5

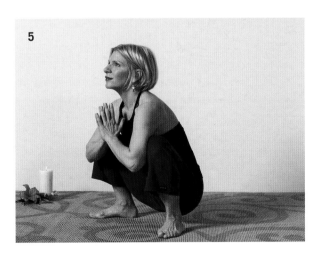

7b

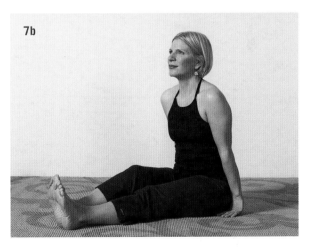

CHAPTER NINE

Unwind

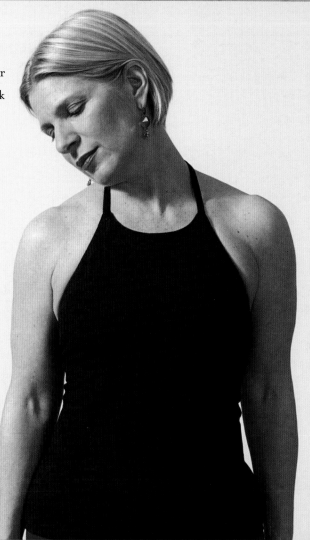

One of the most common spots

to hold on to tension is in the upper back and shoulder area and into the neck. These simple stretches will work best in conjunction with deep, flowing breath. Be conscious of releasing pent-up aggravation and stress with every exhalation. All of the stretches shown can also be performed seated, and you can include any or all of them in your warm-up for more vigorous work or for your regular gym routine.

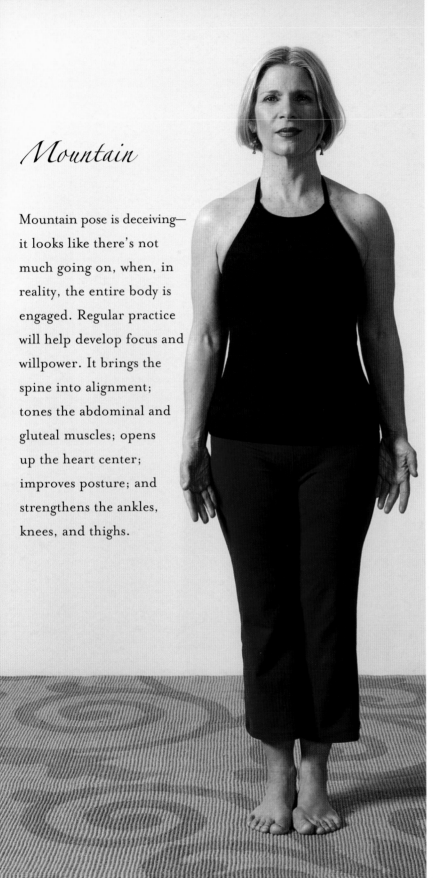

Mountain

Mountain pose is deceiving—it looks like there's not much going on, when, in reality, the entire body is engaged. Regular practice will help develop focus and willpower. It brings the spine into alignment; tones the abdominal and gluteal muscles; opens up the heart center; improves posture; and strengthens the ankles, knees, and thighs.

1. Stand with your feet together, arms at your sides with your palms turned forward. Let your knees face forward and stack them over your ankles. Then stack your hips over your knees, scooping your pelvis forward, letting your tailbone turn downward.

2. Contract your abdominal muscles and lift gently through your heart center. Stack your shoulders over your hips and then draw your shoulder blades together and slide them down your back.

3. Close your eyes and bring your awareness into the soles of your feet, feeling them root into the earth. Inhale and draw the arches of your feet up and lift your kneecaps. Feel the energy moving through your core and into your back, and make a conscious effort to extend your spinal column as you reach out through the crown of your head. (Imagine there's a string attached to the top of your head and someone is pulling on it, causing your bones and muscles to extend upward.)

4. Hold the pose for three to five breaths, continuing to extend your entire body—keeping feet rooted and energy extending through the crown of your head.

Arm Stretch

To gently open up the deltoid muscles.

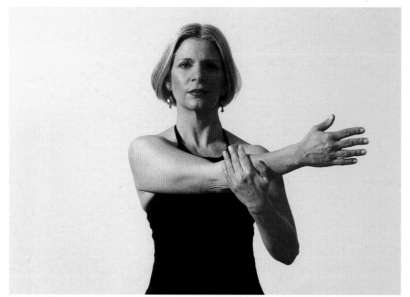

1. Bring your feet to hips' width apart and slightly bend your knees. Cross your right arm in front of your body and cradle your right elbow in your left hand.

2. Gently press your right arm as you drop your shoulder down. Breathe deeply and let go of tension in your arm.

3. Hold for three to five breaths, then repeat to the other side.

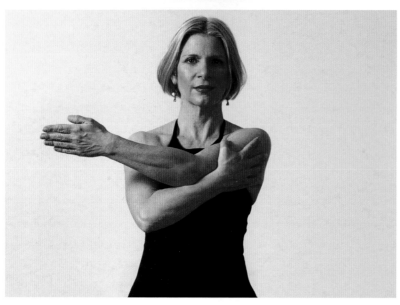

Gentle Side-to-Side Twist

Gently awaken the spine and begin to energize the body.

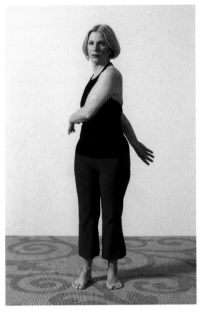

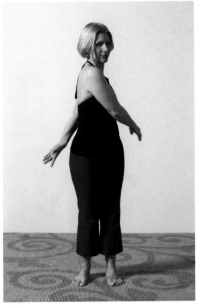

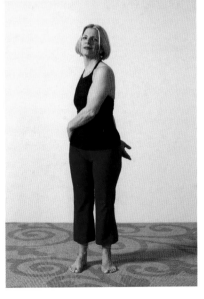

1. Standing with your feet hips' width apart and with a slight bend in your knees, let your arms hang loosely by your sides.

2. Begin to focus on your breath and then slowly begin to twist your torso from side to side.

3. Let your arms be free as you continue to inhale and exhale, moving from left to right.

Ear to Shoulder/Chin to Shoulder

Stretch the neck and let go of tension.

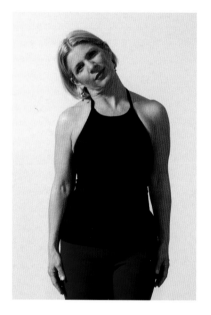 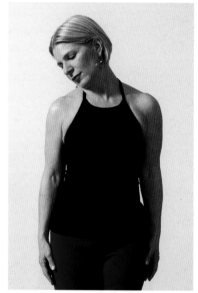 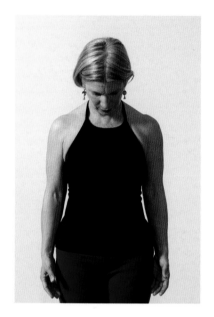

1. Standing with your feet hips' width apart, pull your navel in, and turn your tailbone toward the floor.

2. Keep your shoulder blades drawn together and moving down toward your butt.

3. On an exhalation, gently let your head fall over to the right, letting your right ear drop toward your right shoulder. Don't force it in any way—just let go of the weight of your head and keep your breath flowing evenly.

4. After two or three breaths, turn your chin toward your right shoulder and set your gaze down at the floor. Feel the stretch in the left side of your neck.

5. On an exhalation, drop your chin to center and let the back of your neck extend naturally. Breathe.

6. After two or three breaths roll your head over to the left, letting your left ear fall toward your left shoulder.

7. Hold for two to three breaths, then turn your chin toward your left shoulder and stretch the right side of your neck. Breathe.

8. Continue rolling your head from left to right, then right to left, repeating the sequence two or three times.

9. From center, bring your head upright and go right into the next move.

Shoulder Rolls

Loosen up tight shoulder joints. This should feel like a great shoulder massage!

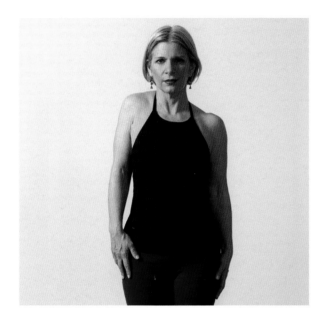 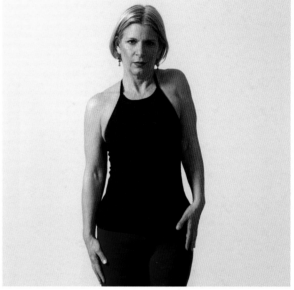

1. Standing with your feet hips' width apart and knees slightly bent, make sure your hips are stacked over your knees and your shoulders over your hips.

2. Let your arms hang loosely by your sides, then move with your breath as you inhale and lift your right shoulder up (like shrugging your shoulder).

3. Exhale and roll it back and down.

4. Repeat to the other side.

5. Continue to roll opposite shoulders up and back for several rounds; then hold at center and reverse the action.

Lateral Flexion

This pose is perfect for opening up the sides of the waist, stretching the obliques as well as the major muscles in the back.

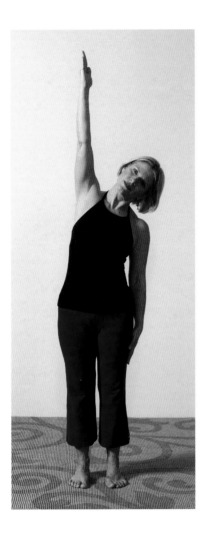

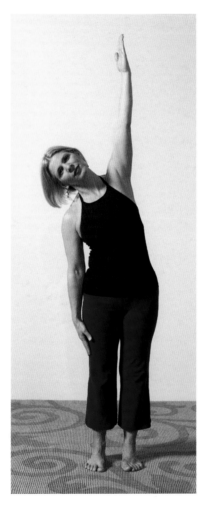

1. Standing with your feet at hips' width, inhale and extend both arms overhead. Exhale and release your left arm down to the left side.

2. Continue reaching through your right fingertips, and on the next inhale, feel your rib cage lifting off the waistline.

3. Exhale and let your body fall over to the left, keeping your right arm extending straight up to the ceiling.

4. Feel your right foot grounding and make sure your torso doesn't cave forward.

5. Breathe into the stretch and be aware of your rib cage expanding.

6. Slowly come back to center and let your left arm come back up overhead. Stretch through all ten fingers for one big breath, then release your right arm down and repeat the sequence to the other side.

Supine Cat

Create space in the upper back and shoulders.

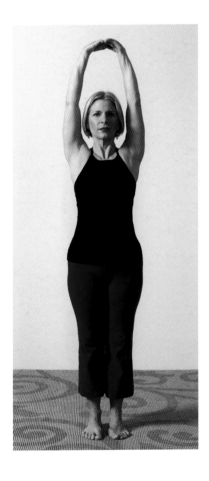 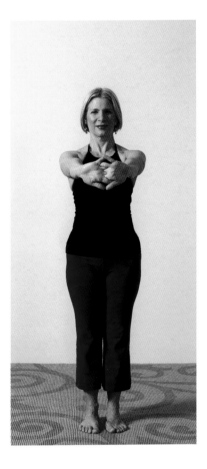

1. Standing with your feet hips' width apart, knees slightly bent, inhale and extend both arms overhead.

2. Interlace your fingers and turn your palms up to face the ceiling.

3. Inhale and extend through your palms, then exhale and slowly lower your arms in front of your body, keeping the extension through your arms.

4. Bring your arms straight ahead, lining up your hands with your heart center.

5. Breathe and round through the shoulders as you press your palms forward. Let your chin drop to your chest.

6. Feel your breath moving into the tight muscles in your upper back and let go.

7. Hold for three to five breaths; then bring your arms back overhead, unclasp the hands, and let them float back down to your sides. Repeat as many times as you'd like.

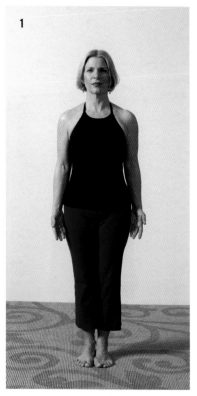

1

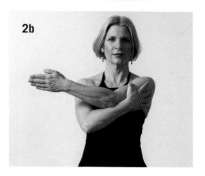

2a

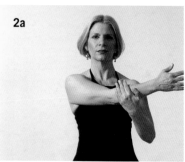

2b

Unwind Sequence

It's 10 P.M. and you're sitting in front of the TV, relaxing for the first time since you got up this morning. I know it will seem like an effort, but I promise it will be worth it—you don't even have to shut off what you're watching—simply start this sequence of postures. You will notice that moving gently actually relaxes you more than not moving. Your mood will improve, too, and your dreams will be restful.

3a

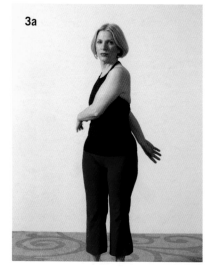

3b

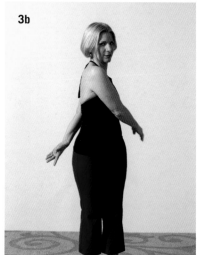

3c

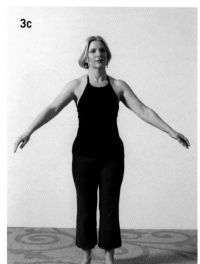

3d

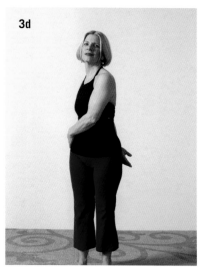

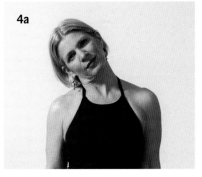

4a

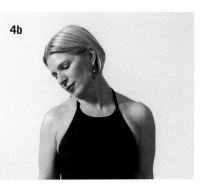

4b

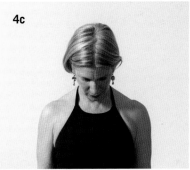

4c

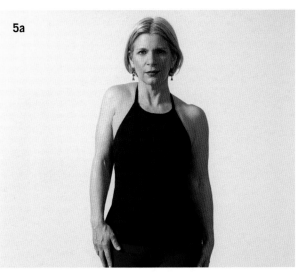

5a

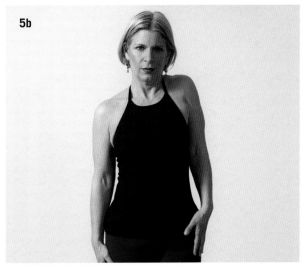

5b

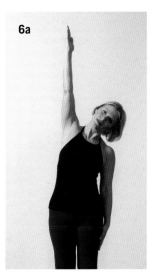

6a

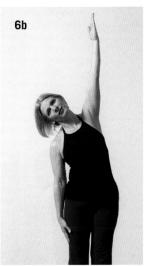

6b

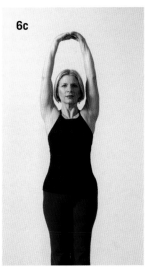

6c

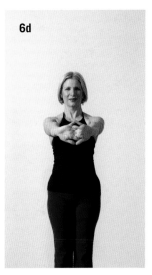

6d

CHAPTER TEN

Warm-up for More Vigorous Work

Use this warm-up whenever

you're feeling low on energy. It will awaken the spine and get the blood and oxygen moving through the arms and legs. Breathe deeply and evenly; notice any tight spots or sore spots and acknowledge them so you can continue to take care and nurture yourself as you move into more challenging postures.

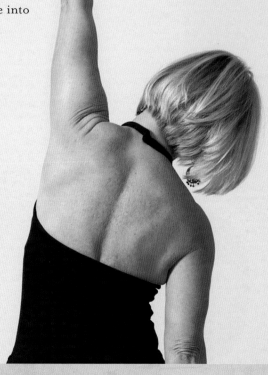

Child's Pose

Begin in Child's Pose to clear the brain and get focused.
Breathe into all the muscles and joints and surrender to the
pose. Don't allow distractions or thoughts in. This is your
chance to assess the body, to calm your mind and prepare for
the work ahead.

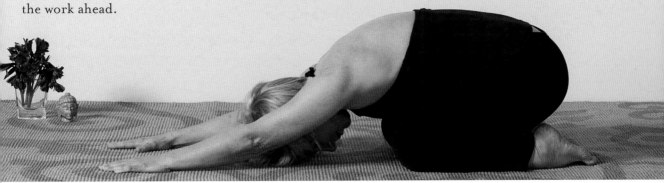

1. Bring yourself onto all fours,
then bring your feet together,
letting your big toes touch, and
keep your knees wide apart.

2. Slide your hips back and let
them rest on your heels, then
extend your arms forward and let
your forehead rest on the floor.

3. Relax and breathe.

Cat Stretch

Increase spinal flexibility; open up the low back, chest, throat, and shoulders while you improve circulation and digestion and stimulate the thyroid and parathyroid glands.

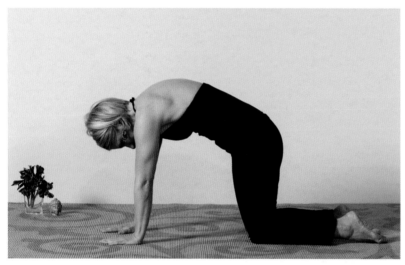

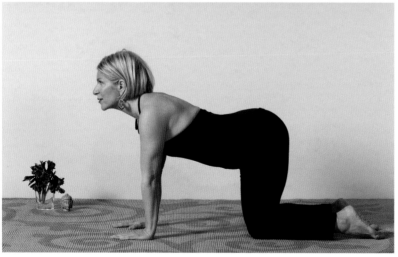

1. Come onto all fours and stack your joints—hips directly over knees, elbows over wrists, shoulders over elbows. Spread your fingers wide and root them into the floor.

2. Make sure your shoulders are away from your ears. No slouching! Draw your shoulder blades together and slide them down your back.

3. Keep your head and neck aligned and set your gaze straight down at the mat.

4. Exhale and draw your navel in, rounding your spine toward the ceiling as you drop your tailbone and lower your head. Breathe deeply.

5. Inhale and let your belly drop as you arch your back, lift your tailbone, and lift your head.

6. Continue exhaling and rounding, inhaling and arching, for several more rounds. Then come back into starting position and either move right into the next pose or rest back in Child's Pose for a few breaths.

Cat Stretch with Extended Leg

Tone the abdominal muscles by modifying Cat Stretch.

1. Come onto all fours and stack your joints—hips directly over knees, elbows over wrists, shoulders over elbows. Spread your fingers wide and root them into the floor.

2. Make sure your shoulders are away from your ears. No slouching! Draw your shoulder blades together and slide them down your back.

3. Keep your head and neck aligned and set your gaze straight down at the mat.

4. Exhale and draw your navel in, rounding the spine toward the ceiling and drawing your right knee in toward your forehead. Use your core strength to hold this position for two or three breaths, then release and extend your right leg straight out behind you as you gently arch your back and lift your head.

5. Repeat the sequence on the same side two more times, then let your right knee come back down and do the whole sequence on the left.

6. Remember to use your breath, keeping the movements flowing and graceful. When you've finished both sides, you can move right into the next pose or rest in Child's Pose.

Spinal Balance

Strengthen all of the back muscles, lengthen the spine, and improve your balance and coordination.

1. Come onto all fours and stack your joints—hips directly over knees, elbows over wrists, shoulders over elbows. Spread your fingers wide and root them into the floor.

2. Make sure your shoulders are away from your ears. No slouching! Draw your shoulder blades together and slide them down your back.

3. Keep your head and neck aligned and set your gaze straight down at the mat.

4. Inhale and extend your right arm and left leg up, parallel to the floor. Your right palm faces the floor; shoulders and hips are squared to the floor.

5. Breathe and feel your arm and leg moving out and away from your core center. Create space and length. Remember to keep your shoulders away from your ears, your head and neck aligned, and your extended knee facing the floor.

6. Exhale and return your right arm and left leg to the floor. Inhale and extend left arm and right leg.

7. Continue extending and releasing opposite arms and legs. Move slowly, with your breath, and create fluid movement for two or three rounds on each side.

8. Come back to starting position and rest back in Child's Pose or go right into the next posture.

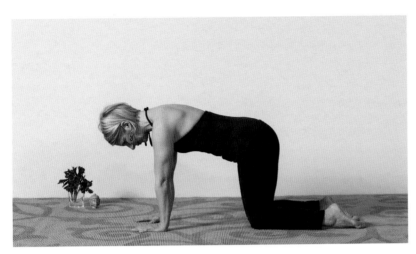

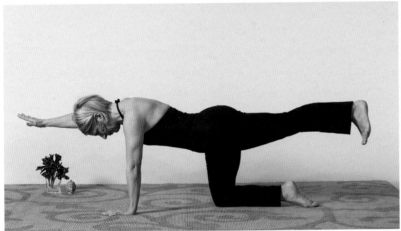

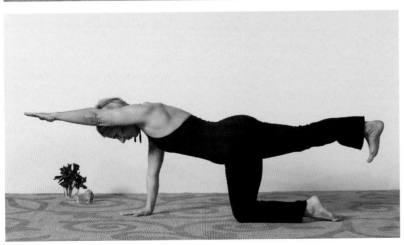

Down Dog (Bicycle Legs)

In a vigorous yoga practice, Down Dog is often used as a transitional pose. On its own it will stretch the palms, chest, back, hamstrings, calves, and feet; strengthen the arms, legs, and torso; and energize the entire body. It can also improve focus and willpower, stimulate the mind, reduce stress, and relieve low back pain. Adding movement to the legs allows the body to warm the leg muscles and further loosen any tightness in the hamstrings and calves.

1. From Child's Pose come up onto all fours. Walk your knees back slightly behind your hips. Place your hands directly under your shoulders and spread your fingers wide, with your middle finger pointing forward.

2. Press down into the roots of your fingers and think about drawing your shoulder blades together, then sliding them down your back.

3. On an inhalation, lift your hips and lengthen through your spine as you roll your shoulders open.

4. Keep a slight bend in your knees and scoop your tailbone even further up, then exhale and straighten your legs, sending your heels toward the floor.

5. Continue to deepen into the pose with every breath, making adjustments and letting your body begin to blossom open.

6. Then bend one knee as you gently press the opposite heel into the floor. Switch legs. Continue to alternate legs, moving into a "bicycle" motion. Repeat five or six reps on each side, then press back into Down Dog.

7. Hold for three to ten breaths, then bend both knees and walk your feet forward, moving into the next pose.

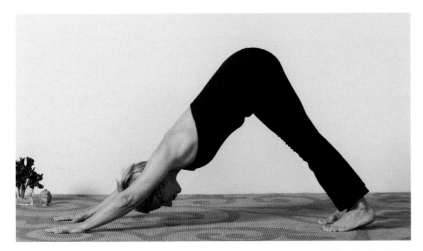

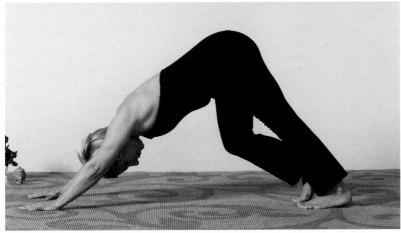

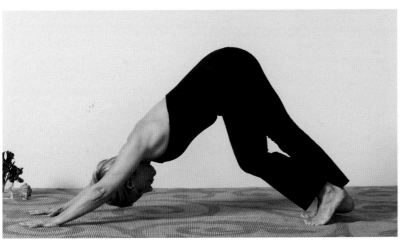

Big Toe Forward Fold

Relieve headaches and insomnia; stimulate the liver, kidneys, and digestive system; stretch the hamstrings and calves; and strengthen the feet, knees, and thighs.

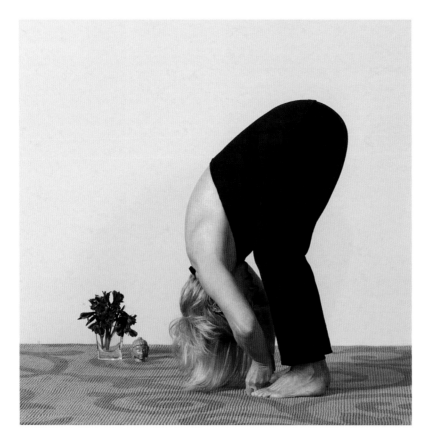

1. If you're starting from Down Dog, bend both knees and walk your feet forward. If you're starting from a standing position, come into Mountain pose but separate the feet to hips' width. Inhale and extend both arms overhead, stretching though your abdominal wall, lifting your rib cage, and sending energy out through all ten fingers.

2. Bend your knees and exhale, letting your arms sweep out to your sides, and float your torso down. Keep the length in your spine as you fold forward.

3. Let your arms hang down and let go of your head and neck. Keep a bend in your knees to protect your low back.

4. Reach down to your toes and wrap the first two fingers of each hand around your big toes as you bend your elbows.

5. Breathe deeply and feel the weight of your head and torso extending your spine with every exhalation.

6. If you want more of a challenge, after at least three full breaths, straighten your knees just a bit as you turn your tailbone up to the sky. Feel your breath moving into your hamstrings and the backs of your knees.

7. After five full breaths in Forward Fold, release your toes and move into the next pose.

Gentle Straddle Stretch

A good stretch for the waist, inner thighs, and lower back. It will also reduce stress and help relieve headache or sinus problems.

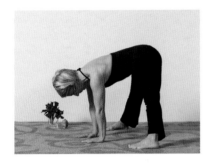 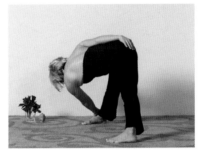 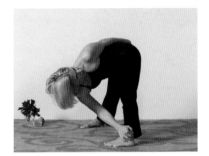

1. From Forward Fold, heel-toe feet apart (anywhere from three to five feet) into straddle position with your feet parallel.

2. Place your hands on the floor directly under your shoulders. Keep your spine long and flat.

3. Walk your hands over to your right leg and hold onto your right ankle with your left hand.

4. Bend your elbow, exhale, and release your spine, pulling your torso a little closer to your leg if you can. Don't force the stretch.

Breathe into it and feel tension melting away on your breath. Hold for three to five breaths, then slowly walk your hands back to center.

5. Take a breath, and on an exhalation, walk your hands over to the left and repeat the sequence.

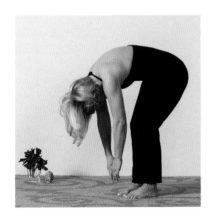

Transition
When you've stretched both sides, come back to center with your hands under your shoulders. Heel-toe feet together and press down into your feet as you draw your navel in and roll up to standing.

Warm-up for More Vigorous Work Sequence

By warm-up, I am not suggesting that this sequence isn't a workout in itself!
It can certainly be used as a series on its own. I'm only describing it as a warm-up
because it moves the spine in all direction, thus allowing it to be ready to do
tougher moves. But feel free to use this sequence at any time during the day to
ease any tension you feel in all areas of your back.

1

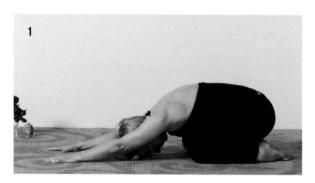

3a

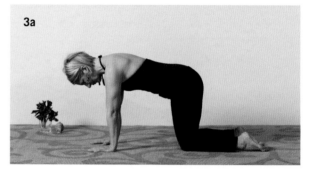

2a

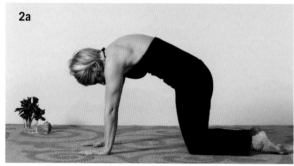

3b

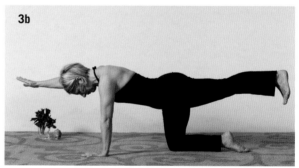

2b

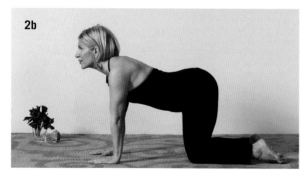

3c

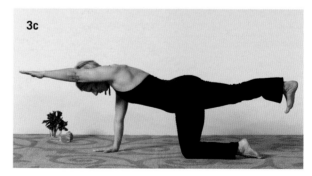

4a

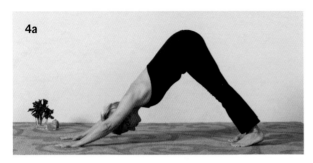

4b

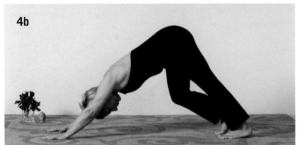

4c

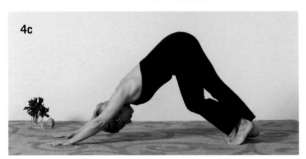

5

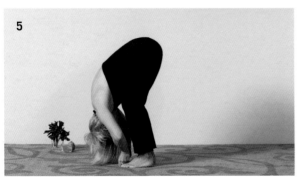

6a

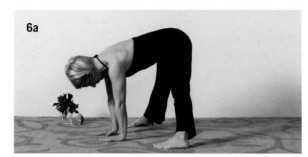

6b

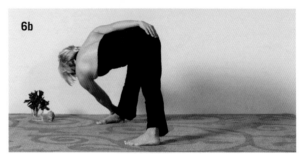

6c

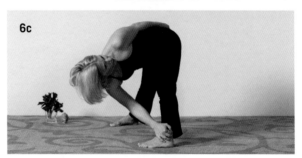

6d

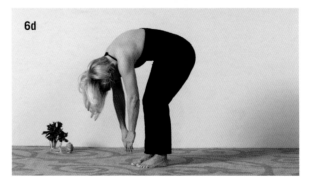

CHAPTER ELEVEN

Strengthen the Lower Back, Hips, and Glutes

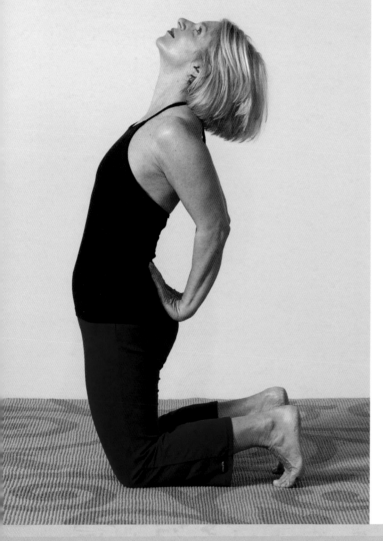

Build a strong foundation for your whole body, especially your back, by strengthening the powerful muscles in your lower body. These standing postures build stamina and muscular endurance, add length to your spine, and will help relieve symptoms of sciatica.

Mountain

Mountain pose is deceiving—it looks like there's not much going on, when, in reality, the entire body is engaged. Regular practice will help develop focus and willpower. It brings the spine into alignment; tones the abdominal and gluteal muscles; opens up the heart center; improves posture; and strengthens the ankles, knees, and thighs.

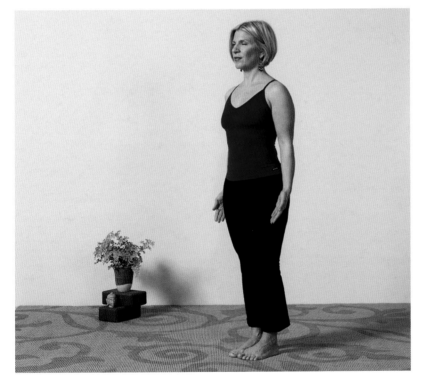

2. Contract your abdominal muscles and lift gently through your heart center. Stack your shoulders over your the hips and then draw your shoulder blades together and slide them down your back.

3. Close your eyes and bring your awareness into the soles of your feet, feeling them root into the earth. Inhale and draw the arches of your feet up and lift your kneecaps. Feel the energy moving through your core and into your back, and make a conscious effort to extend your spinal column as you reach out through the crown of your head. (Imagine there's a string attached to the top of your head and someone is pulling on it, causing your bones and muscles to extend upward.)

4. Hold the pose for three to five breaths, continuing to extend your entire body, keeping feet rooted and energy extending through the crown of your head.

1. Stand with your feet together, arms at your sides with your palms turned forward. Let your knees face forward and stack them over your ankles. Then stack your hips over your knees, scooping your pelvis forward, letting your tailbone turn downward.

Warrior 1

Tap into your warrior spirit and find courage and confidence as you build endurance, stretch the hips and shoulders, strengthen your legs, stimulate digestion, and develop willpower.

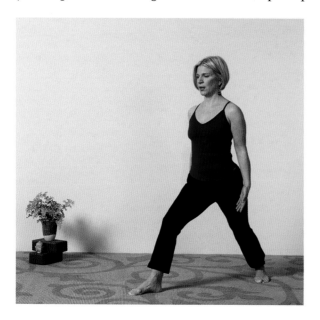 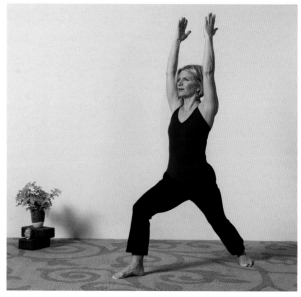

1. From Mountain pose, take a step back with your left foot and angle your toes so that they are turned out slightly. Look down at your feet and check to make sure that the heel of your front foot is lining up with the heel of your back foot.

2. Turn your hips and shoulders to face the front. Think about lifting the inside of your left ankle so that the outside edge of that foot connects to the floor.

3. Inhale and sweep your arms overhead, reaching through all ten fingers. Slide your shoulders down, away from your ears.

4. Exhale and bend your right knee as you sink into a lunge. Make sure your knee doesn't move forward over your toes. It should remain aligned with your ankle throughout the pose.

5. Each time you inhale, extend further up through your fingers, and each time you exhale, sink deeper into the lunge. Hold for three to five breaths, then come up slowly, release your arms, and step your left foot back up to your right.

6. Repeat the sequence to the other side.

Warrior 2

Open up your heart center and increase lung capacity. Stretch your shoulders and hips, lengthen the spine, stimulate circulation and the mind, strengthen the legs, and build endurance with the proud Warrior 2 pose.

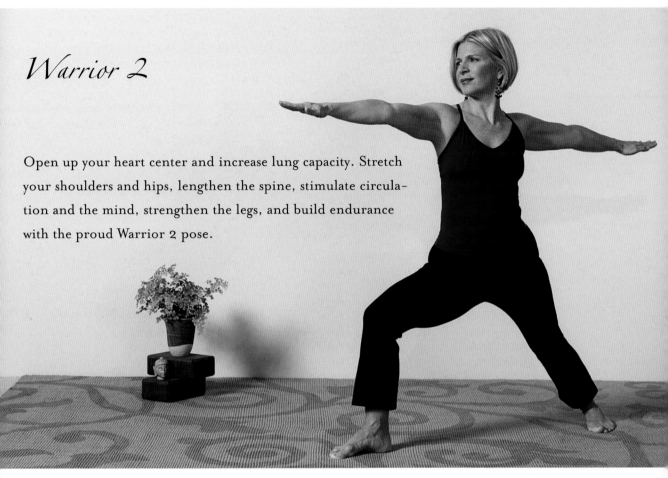

1. Standing in Mountain pose, step your feet wide apart with your feet parallel. Inhale and extend your arms out to your sides.

2. Turn your right toes to the right side, and keep your left toes parallel or slightly turned in.

3. Turn your head to gaze over the middle finger of your right hand.

4. Exhale and bend your right knee as you lower into a lunge. Keep your knee directly over your ankle. Soften your shoulders and draw your navel in. Imagine there is someone standing in front of and behind you, holding on to your fingertips and stretching you in opposite directions.

5. With each inhalation, extend through your arms, and with each exhalation, sink deeper. Hold for three to five breaths, then slowly straighten your right leg.

6. Keeping your arms extended, turn your toes in the opposite direction—pointing your left toes straight and angling the right. Repeat the sequence and return to Mountain pose or continue to the next pose.

Triangle

Triangle is also called Happy Pose because it opens up your heart center, allowing you to give and receive joy and love! It also relieves stress and sciatica, which may make you feel happy too, and it lengthens your spine, stabilizes your torso and your legs, and builds focus.

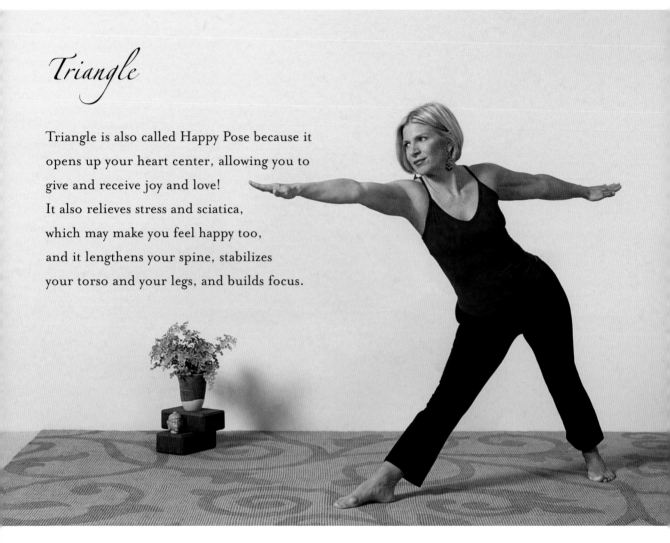

1. You can go right into Triangle from Warrior 2, or you can begin in Mountain.

2. Standing with your feet wide apart and the feet parallel, turn your right toes to the right side and keep your left toes parallel or slightly turned in.

3. Inhale and extend your arms out to your sides, then turn your head to gaze over the middle finger of your right hand.

4. Engage the muscles in your legs and feel your feet rooted to the floor. Inhale and extend your right fingertips over your right toes—as

if someone were pulling your fingers. Keep your torso long.

5. Exhale as you windmill your arms down, letting your right hand rest at some point on your right leg, or, if you're more flexible, place your fingertips on the floor next to your right foot.

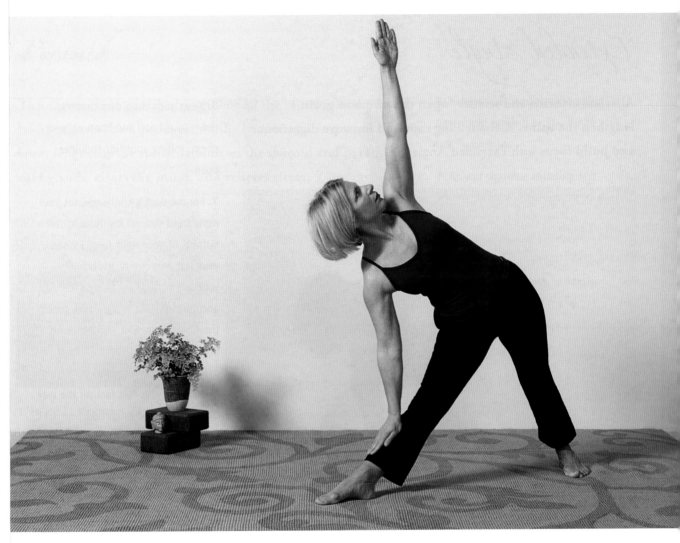

6. Your body should be moving laterally—imagine being pressed between two panes of glass. If you find your torso is caving forward, ease up a little until you can stack your lungs and your ribs.

7. Gaze up at your left thumb or, if your neck hurts, look down at your big toe. Breathe deeply—keep making adjustments and notice the changes occurring in your body as you sink deeper into the pose.

8. Hold for three to five breaths, then inhale and let your extended (left) arm pull you back up.

9. Turn your toes in the opposite direction and repeat the sequence to the other side, then move into the next pose.

Straddle Twist

Believe it or not, the wider your legs are in this pose, the easier it will be. This is a wonderful strengthener for your feet, ankles, knees, inner thighs, and lower back. It will also tone your abdominal muscles, build focus and willpower, reduce stress, and even help relieve sinus problems.

1. Stand with your feet together, arms at your sides with your palms turned forward. Let your knees face forward and stack them over your ankles. Then stack your hips over your knees, scooping your pelvis forward, letting your tailbone turn downward.

2. Inhale and extend both arms overhead, stretching though your abdominal wall, lifting your rib cage, and sending energy out through all ten fingers.

3. Bend your knees and exhale, letting your arms sweep out to the sides, and float your torso down. Keep the length in your spine as you fold forward.

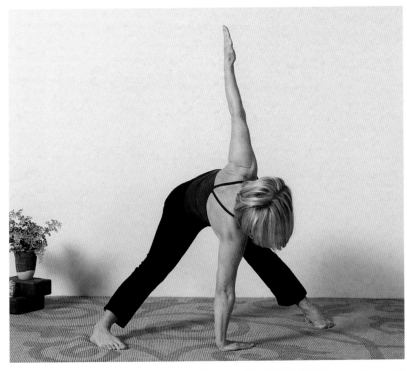

4. Heel-toe feet apart (anywhere from three to five feet) into a straddle position and keep your feet parallel or let the heels be a little wider than the toes.

5. Place your hands on the floor directly under your shoulders. Keep your spine long and flat. Shift the weight of your body back.

6. Place your right hand directly under your heart center and turn your hand so the pinky side faces out.

7. Bring your left hand onto the left hip. Inhale and roll your left shoulder up to the ceiling, turning your entire torso from the hips.

8. Extend your left fingertips up toward the ceiling and gaze up at your thumb.

9. Keep your wrist, elbow, and shoulder of the left arm in one long line. Press into the floor and twist your torso deeper.

10. Hold for three to five breaths, then release, come back to center, switch hands, and repeat to the other side.

11. Heel-toe your feet back together, press through your feet, pull your navel in, and roll up.

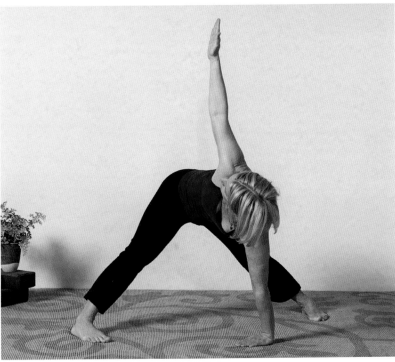

Strengthen the Lower Back, Hips, and Glutes Sequence

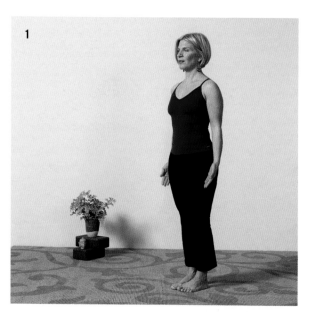

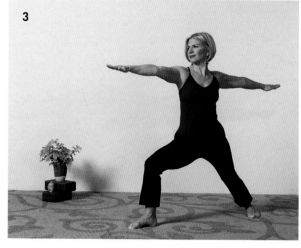

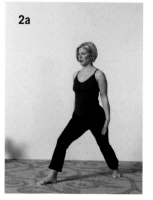

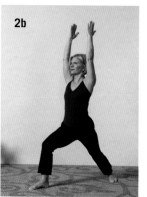

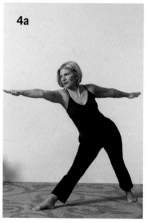

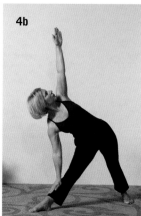

5

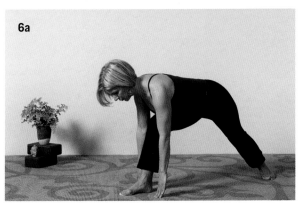

6a

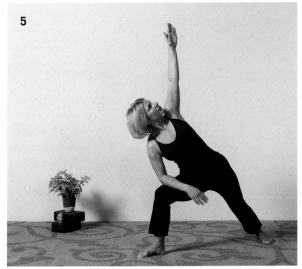

6b

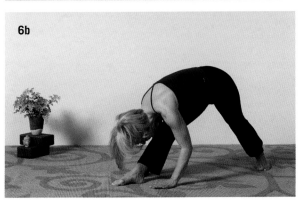

7a

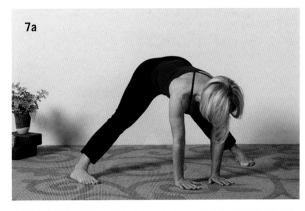

7b

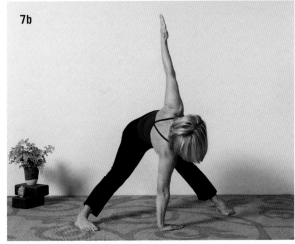

7c

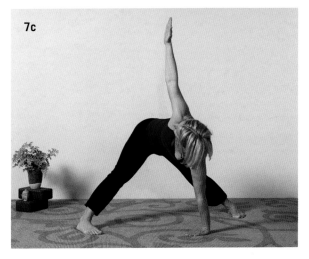

CHAPTER TWELVE

Abdominal Strength

Strengthening the abdominal muscles or

core center will provide essential support for your back as well as for
your internal organs. The abdominal work in yoga is especially good for
your back because the moves are practiced slowly, always with your
breath, and always with awareness. Start out by performing each of these
movements for three to six repetitions and work your way up to as many
reps as possible as you get stronger. You can never do too many—the end
result will be not only a stronger back and core, but a flat, toned belly.

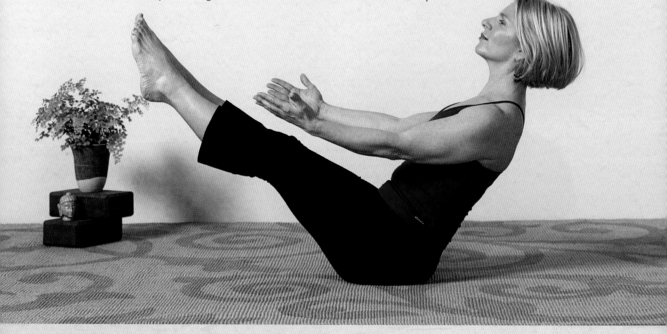

Basic Yoga Crunch

Crunches improve overall strength and tone your torso. Make sure you maintain a neutral spine throughout the movement and keep your knees bent to protect your back. (When you get stronger, you can extend your legs.)

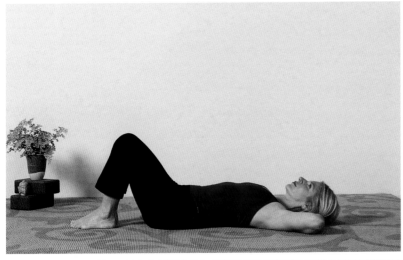

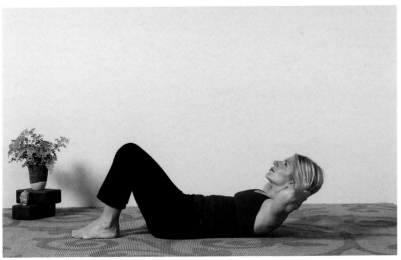

1. Lie on your back with your knees bent and feet flat on the floor.

2. Tilt your pelvis so that your low back and torso come into a neutral position.

3. Cradle your head as you keep your elbows extended out to both sides. Exhale; draw your navel in; and lift your head, neck, and shoulders off the floor. Maintain the contraction and breathe. This is your starting position.

4. Exhale, lift your heart center up to the ceiling, and hold for one or two breaths. Don't strain your neck, and don't let your abdominal muscles pop out.

5. Inhale and release to the starting position. Continue lifting on the exhales and lowering on the inhales for as many reps as feel good to you.

6. When you've finished your reps, let your knees fall open, bring the soles of your feet together, and rest.

7. Get centered, find the rhythm of your breath, and go right into the next move.

Oblique Crunch

By rotating your torso and keeping it still, you will stabilize your lower body, allowing you to isolate the oblique muscles that run along the sides of your body.

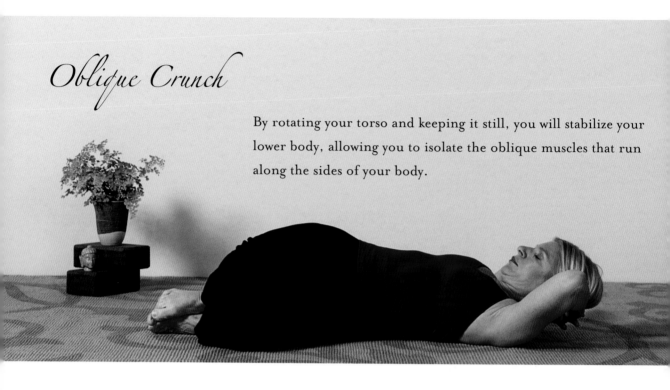

1. Lie on your back with bent knees and your feet flat on the floor.

2. Exhale and drop both legs over to the left, keeping your heart center facing straight up and both shoulders on the floor.

3. Bring your hands behind your head, with elbows extended out to your sides.

4. Exhale and lift your head and shoulders up off the floor. This is your starting position. Breathe.

5. Exhale and lift your torso straight up to the ceiling. Work deep. You

should be able to feel this movement in your right side.

6. Hold for one or two breaths then inhale and come back to starting.

7. Repeat three to six times; then bring your legs back to center, take a few breaths, and on an exhalation, drop your legs over to the right.

8. Repeat the sequence to the other side, and when you're finished, let your knees fall open, bring the soles of your feet together, and rest for a few breaths before you go into the next move.

Double Leg Lift

This move requires focus and determination. It will strengthen your abdominal muscles, which will, in turn, support your low back. Take care not to swing your legs, and remember to breathe. You can modify the pose by letting one foot remain on the floor. With regular practice, leg lifts will help alleviate lower back pain.

1. Lie on your back and bring your spine into neutral alignment. Let your arms rest alongside your body or, to keep your low back on the floor, place both hands under your low back for extra support.

2. Inhale and extend your legs straight up to the ceiling, then flex both feet, pushing energy out through your heels. Feel all the muscles of your legs activating.

3. Pull your navel in toward your spine and extend your tailbone along the floor.

4. On an exhalation, slowly lower your legs to a count of ten. The lower you get, the harder it will become. Continue to push out through your heels, and feel every muscle in your legs activating (this will tone your legs). Stay focused and keep your core strong.

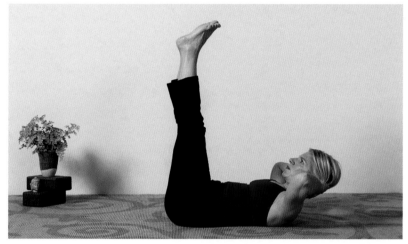

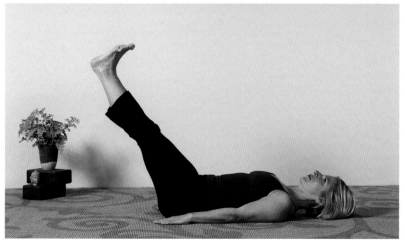

continued on next page >

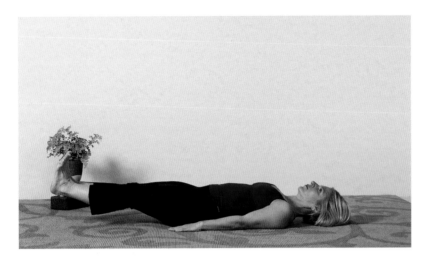

5. As soon as your heels touch the floor, inhale and bring your legs back up. You can repeat two more times, or hug your knees in and roll from side to side to release your back.

6. Come back to center, cross your legs at the ankles, hold on to your big toes, and rock up to a seated position so you can move on to the next pose.

Transition

Rock and roll up to a comfortable seated position and rest for a few breaths.

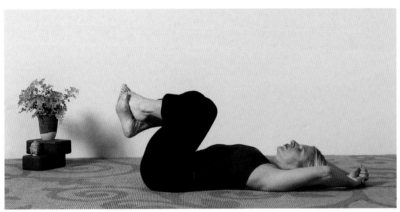

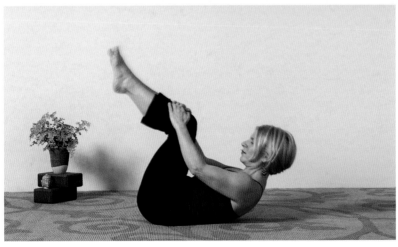

Modified Boat

Boat pose not only builds a strong core, but it also lengthens the spine and neck; strengthens the legs, hips, groin, and abdominal muscles; improves balance, posture, and digestion; and opens the throat and shoulders.

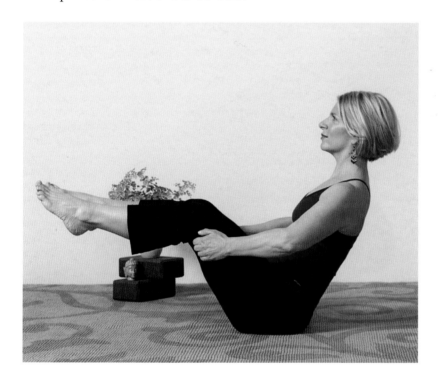

1. Sitting on the floor, move the fleshy part of your butt away from your sitting bones. Feel your connection to the floor.

2. Extend your spine up and reach out through the crown of your head.

3. Bend both knees and wrap your hands around the backs of your thighs, then lean back and balance between your sitting bones and tailbone.

4. Draw your navel in, keeping your core strong and engaged. Exhale and extend your legs at an upward angle as you stretch your arms forward.

5. Squeeze your shoulder blades together and lift your heart as you open your chest.

6. Hold for three to five breaths or as long as you can, then slowly release and roll back down to the floor.

Bridge

Bridge pose will awaken the spine and open up the belly, releasing tight abdominal muscles. It improves flexibility in the shoulders and spine; stimulates the thyroid and parathyroid glands; increases lung capacity; and relieves high blood pressure, stress, and asthma.

1. Bend your knees and place your feet flat on the floor, parallel and hips' width apart. Rest your arms alongside your body with your palms flat.

2. Scoop your tailbone forward and rest your low back as close to the floor as is comfortable. Pull your navel in, keeping your core center strong.

3. On an inhalation, press into the soles of your feet and lift your hips up. Use your glutes to help lift.

4. Feel the weight of the body shifting toward your shoulders, then draw your shoulder blades together, bring your arms underneath your body, and interlace your fingers.

5. Hold for two or three breaths, then draw your navel in and slowly lower, tucking your pelvis as you roll through each vertebra.

6. As soon as your tailbone touches the floor, let your knees fall open, place the soles of your feet together, and rest.

7. Bring your knees back together and hug them into your chest, then go into the next move.

Plow

Strengthen the spine, stretch the shoulders, stimulate the thyroid and parathyroid glands, relieve backache, and calm the mind with Plow. Just be sure to keep the head and neck in alignment and don't turn your head.

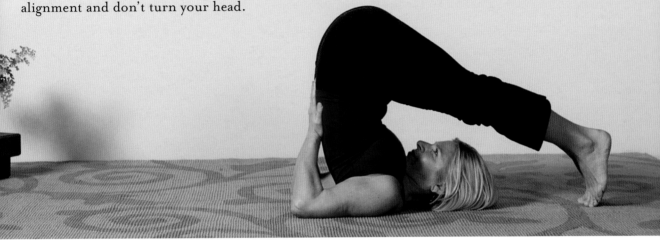

1. Lie on your back with your knees pulled into your chest and your hands cradling your hips.

2. Inhale and lift your hips up, then exhale and extend your legs overhead.

3. Keep your hands on your back for support. If your toes are touching the floor, then you can extend your arms and interlace your fingers.

4. Breathe into the pose. Feel your neck elongate as you reach through the crown of your head. Melt your shoulders into the floor and feel the warmth of your breath moving into your cervical spine.

5. Hold for three to five breaths; then bring your hands onto your back and slowly roll down out of the pose.

6. As soon as your tailbone touches the floor, let your knees fall open, place the soles of your feet together, and rest.

7. Bring your knees back together and extend your legs along the floor, then go into the next move.

Fish

A wonderfully restorative pose, Fish strengthens the muscles of the upper back, neck, and shoulders; helps relieve asthma and stress; improves your voice, digestion, and posture; and energizes the mind.

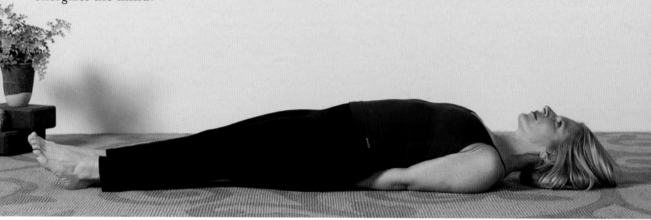

1. Extend your legs along the floor and bring them together, as if they were tied or glued together.

2. Roll your hips from side to side and slide your arms underneath your body. Make sure that your elbows are under your torso and that you're sitting on your hands with your palms facing the floor.

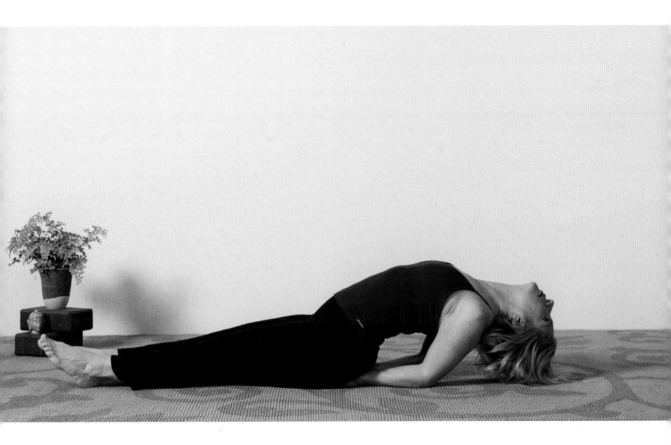

3. Inhale, press into your elbows as you lift your chest and let your head drop back. Exhale and release the crown of your head to the floor.

4. Hold for three to ten breaths, letting your lungs expand and your throat open.

5. Slowly lower your back down and hug your knees.

6. Drop your feet to the floor; then let your knees fall open as you bring the soles of your feet together and rest.

Abdominal Strength Sequence

Strong abs can do more to help cure back pain than almost anything else (except perhaps losing excess weight). And you don't have to do traditional abdominal exercises or buy one piece of equipment to see—and feel—a real difference in your abs. But you will quickly feel a difference in your posture, because strong abs can make you walk, stand, and sit taller than you ever have before.

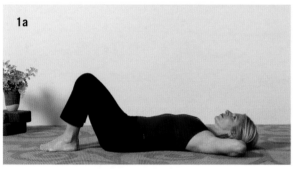

1a

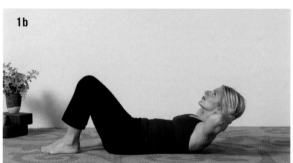

1b

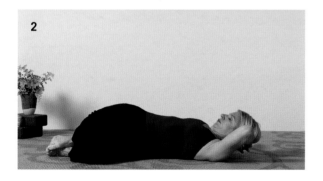

2

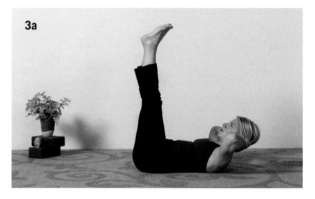

3a

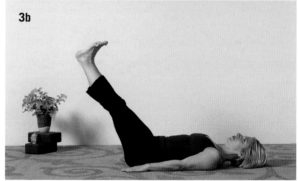

3b

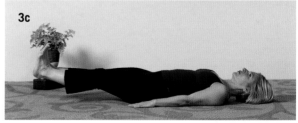

3c

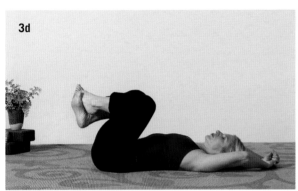

3d

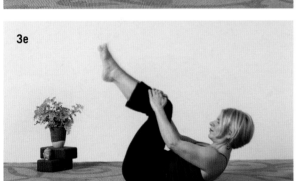

3e

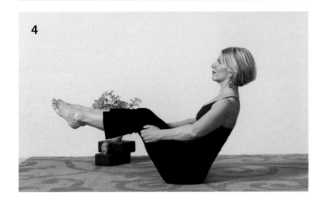

4

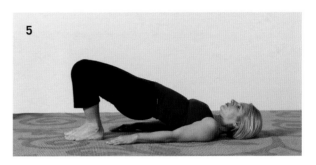

5

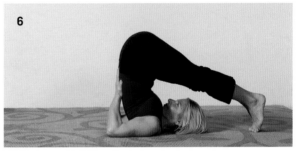

6

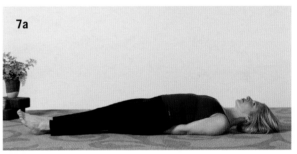

7a

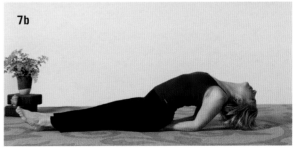

7b

CHAPTER THIRTEEN

Modified Sun Series

Sun Series, or Sun Salutation, can be

performed anytime, but it's especially good at sunrise or sunset or whenever you need to take your energy level up a notch. You can do the series slowly or, for a more aerobic practice, do it quickly. Whichever way you choose, be sure to flow consciously and always with your breath. You'll want to create warmth and energy, but don't move so fast that you lose control of your movements. Do it as a self-contained practice or attach it before and/or after any of the other routines.

Sun Series will energize, tone, and strengthen all of the muscles and organs of your body.

Mountain

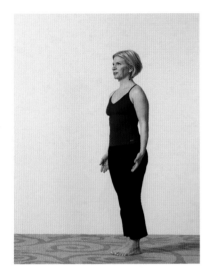

Arms overhead

hands to low back for gentle backbend

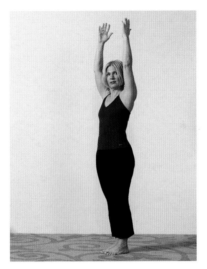

Arms overhead

hands to namaste, release to heart, fold forward

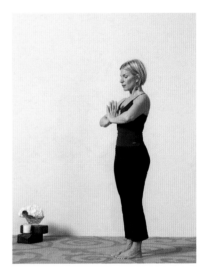

Begin in Mountain, with your arms at your sides and eyes closed. Feel your feet ground into the earth; contract your leg, gluteal, and abdominal muscles. Find your breath and get into a natural rhythm. Keep your breath moving in and out through your nose for the entire practice. Let your shoulders slide down your back and extend your spine from your tailbone all the way up and out through the crown of your head.

Inhale and sweep your arms overhead, spreading your fingers wide and keeping your shoulders down. Take yourself into a gentle backbend—just to the point where you feel your low back activating.

Exhale as you bring your hands to prayer, or namaste, and bring them to your heart center. Inhale, then exhale and, bending your knees, fold forward. Keep a deep bend in your knees and let your torso rest on your thighs—this will help support your spine and allow you to stretch further while protecting your back. Release the weight of your head and shoulders. Let the weight extend your spine. Breathe. Feel your rib cage expanding out to your sides, and with every exhalation, let go of tension, aggravation, and any worries.

Hands on shins

lift heart, flatten back

Bend knees, step left foot back to Lunge

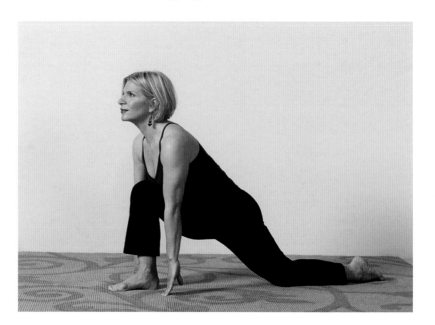

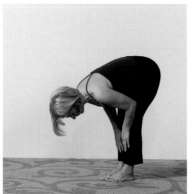

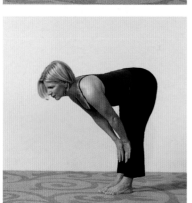

Bring your hands onto your shins and inhale as you lift your heart and flatten your back.

You should feel the stretch into your hamstrings. Exhale and fold forward.

Bend your knees deeply, bringing your hands onto the floor. Inhale and step back with your left foot, coming into a lunge on your right. Drop your left knee down and turn to the top of your left foot, shifting off your kneecap, making sure that your left hip is forward of your left knee and your right knee is directly over your right ankle. Exhale and release your left hip, then inhale and press your fingertips to the floor as you lift through your heart center.

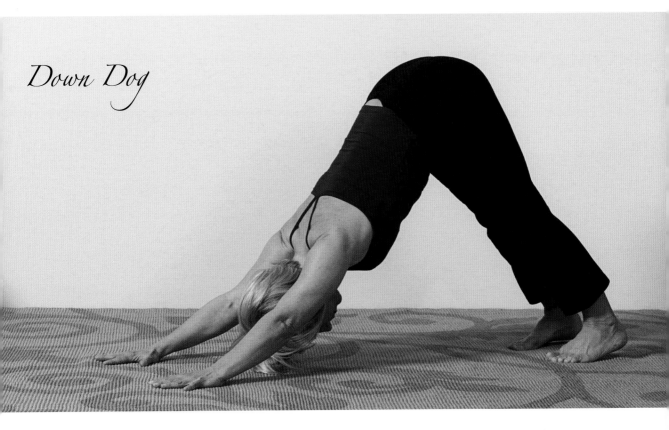

Down Dog

Step your right foot back to your left, then curl your toes under, press into the balls of your feet, and exhale as you press up into Down Dog. Push into the roots of your fingers and spread them wide; slide your shoulders down toward your butt. Lift your kneecaps and press the front of your thighs into the back; then send your heels toward the floor (they don't have to touch, just send them in that direction). Inhale and exhale. With each full breath, stretch deeper into the pose. If Down Dog feels too challenging, you can come into Puppy Pose (see page 138).

Modification: Puppy Pose

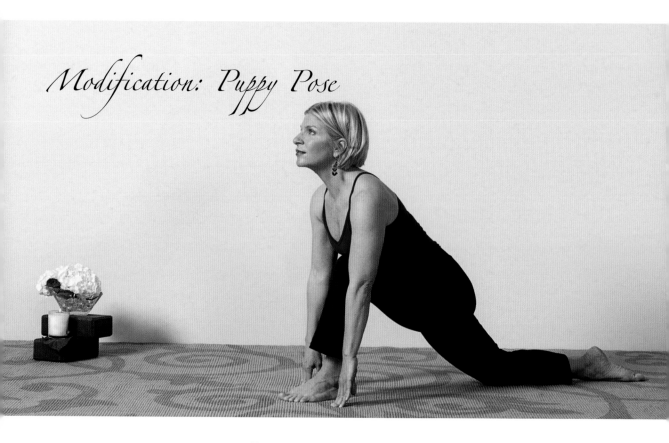

From the lunge, step your right foot
back and place your right knee on
the floor. Make sure your knees are
hips' width apart, then exhale as
you press into the roots of your
fingers and shift your hips back,
extending your spine and your
arms. Don't let your butt drop down
to your heels—keep it lifted and
breathe into the stretch. It should
feel so good!

Drop knees, chest, chin to floor

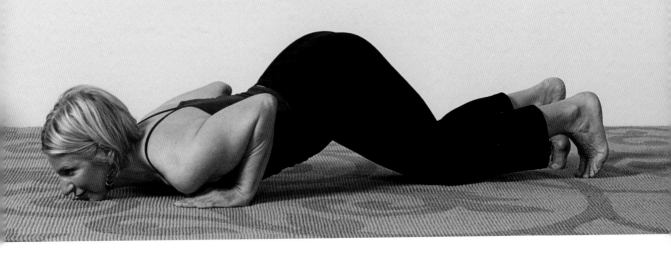

From Down Dog exhale and drop your knees, chest, and chin to the floor. Keep your arms close to your body and your shoulders sliding down your back. Lower the pelvis.

Or, fom Puppy Pose, drop your chest and chin down, keeping your arms close to your body and your shoulders sliding down your back.

Sweep through, lift to Half Cobra

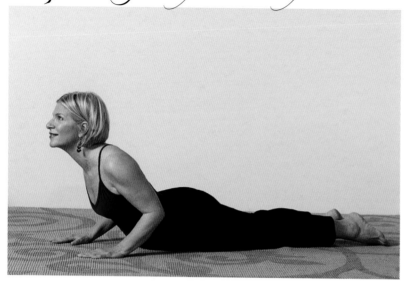

Place the tops of your feet on the floor. Inhale and lift through your heart center, keeping your arms close as you press into your pelvis and the tops of your feet. Feel your low back energizing and squeeze your shoulder blades together as you lift your hands two or three inches off the floor. Breathe!

Push to all fours

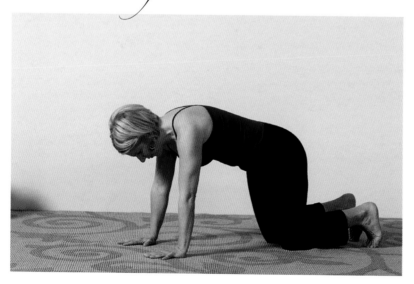

Make sure your hands are under your shoulders, then exhale and press up onto all fours.

Press back to Down Dog

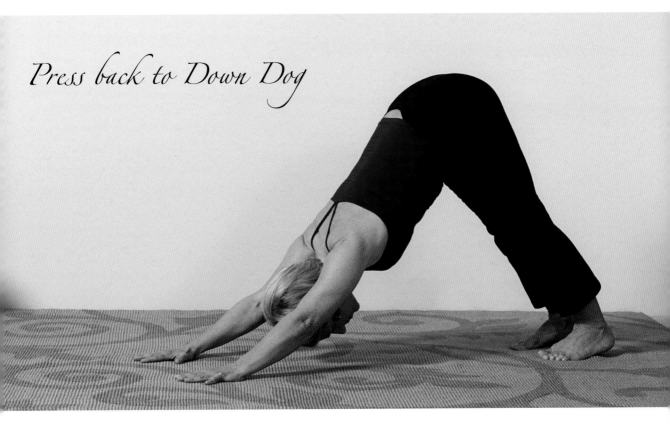

Curl your toes under, slide the
knees back a few inches, spread
your fingers wide, push into the
balls of your feet, and exhale as you
press up into Down Dog (or modify
with Puppy Pose).

Step through with left foot to Lunge

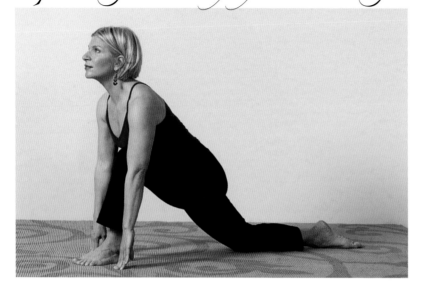

Look up at your hands, inhale, and step your left foot through your arms, placing it on the floor between your hands. You may need to take several steps or perhaps help your foot into the lunge by guiding it into position with your hand. Drop your right knee down and turn to the top of your right foot, shifting off your kneecap, making sure that your right hip is forward of your right knee and your left knee is directly over your left ankle. Exhale and release your right hip, then inhale and press your fingertips to the floor as you lift through your heart center.

Come back to Forward Fold

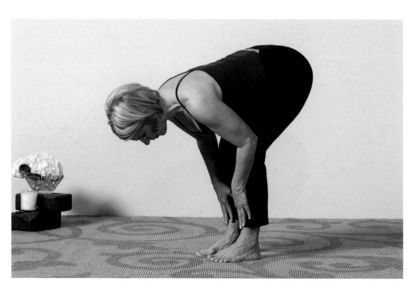

Inhale as you press into your left foot and bring your right foot up to meet your left, returning to Forward Fold. Keep a deep bend in your knees and let your torso rest on your thighs—this will help support your spine and allow you to stretch further while protecting your back. Release the weight of your head and shoulders. Let the weight extend your spine. Breathe. Feel your rib cage expanding out to your sides and with every exhalation, let go of tension, aggravation, and any worries.

Lift heart

Inhale back up to Mountain

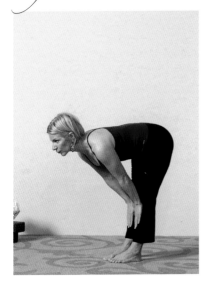

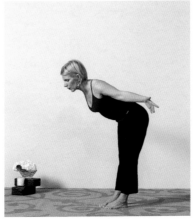

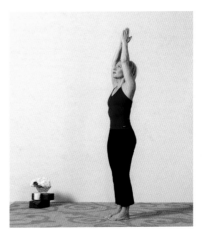

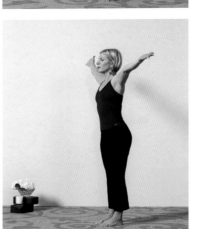

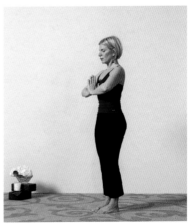

Bring your hands onto your shins and inhale as you lift your heart and flatten your back.

You should feel the stretch into your hamstrings. Exhale and fold forward.

Draw your navel in and inhale as you send your arms out to your sides and lift your heart, bringing yourself back up and into Mountain. Remain in Mountain for a few

breaths, letting yourself observe the changes and energy shifts that occurred in your body. When you're ready, repeat for at least two more rounds or for as many as six.

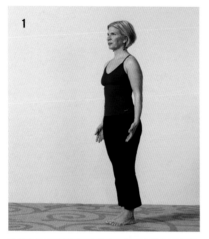

1

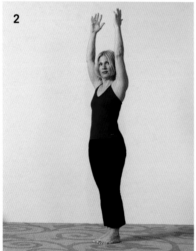

2

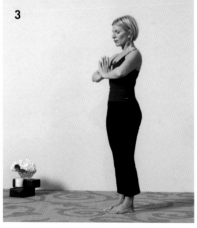

3

Modified Sun Series

The Sun Series begins many yoga classes and many yogi's days. You can use this sequence before any workout to warm up—the modifications make it easier, but no less effective. You can do the entire series as many times as you want to get an aerobic benefit, too.

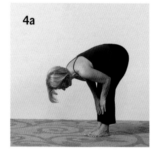

4a

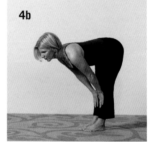

4b

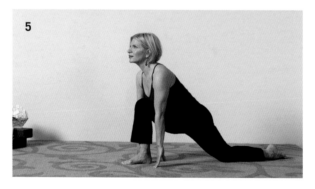

5

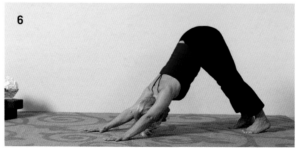

6

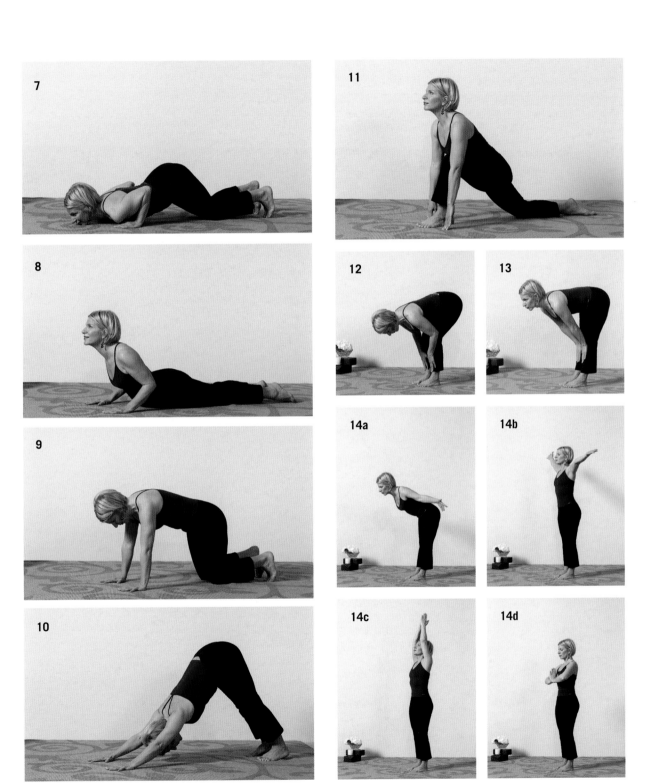

CHAPTER FOURTEEN

Using Props

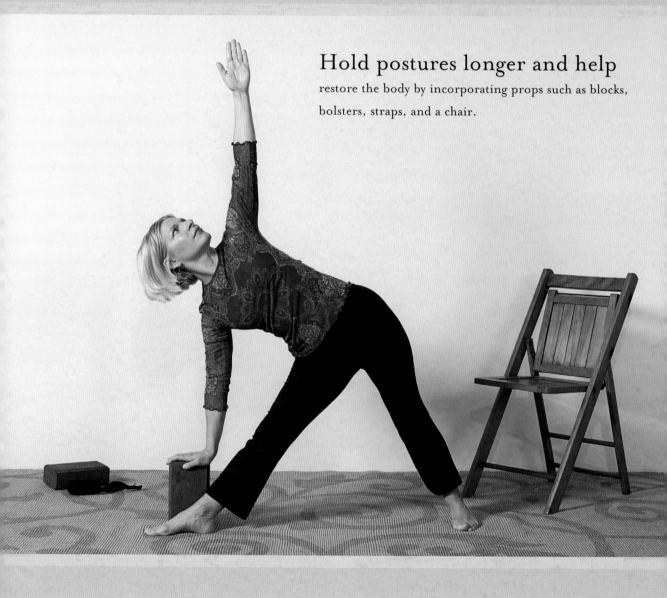

Hold postures longer and help

restore the body by incorporating props such as blocks,
bolsters, straps, and a chair.

Child's Pose

Child's Pose will clear the brain and help to get you focused. If you have very tight shoulder, hip, or knee joints, you might need to modify to help ease your body into the stretch. Remember to breathe into all the muscles and joints and surrender to the pose. Don't allow distractions or thoughts in.

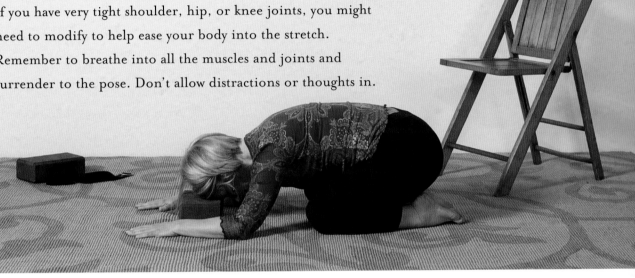

1. Bring yourself onto all fours, then bring your feet together, letting your big toes touch, and keep your knees wide apart. Place a yoga block in between your hands.

2. Slide your hips back and let them rest on your heels, then extend your arms forward and let your forehead rest on the block.

3. Relax and breathe.

Seated Forward Fold

A counterpose to backbends, Seated Forward Fold rests and mas-sages your heart, soothes your adrenal glands, tones your internal organs, activates a sluggish liver, and improves digestion. It also stretches your spine, hamstrings, and calves; calms your nervous system; and alleviates high blood pressure. If you have very tight hamstrings or back pain, modify the pose using a strap.

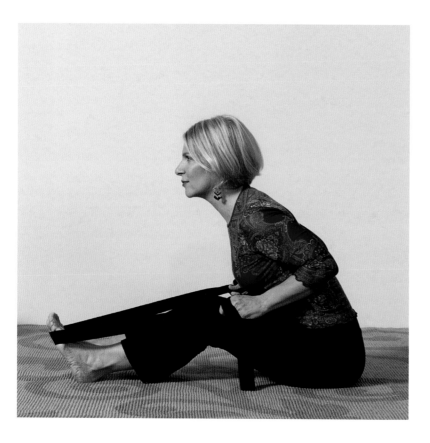

1. Sit with your legs extended along the floor, straight out in front of you. Move the fleshy part of your butt away from your sitting bones and feel your connection to the floor.

2. Bend your knees and place a yoga strap around the soles of your feet, holding one end in each hand.

3. Inhale and extend your spine—sending energy all the way up and out through the crown of your head. Wrap the ends of the strap around your hands.

4. Exhale and hinge at your hips, letting your torso fall forward. Bend your elbows and use the strap to pull your torso further; maintain a straight spine. If you feel your back rounding, ease off and stay at the point where you can hold a straight spine.

5. Breathe and let go of tension as you surrender to your breath and to gravity. Hold for three to ten breaths, then slowly ease back up. Don't force the stretch—wherever you are is exactly where you should be.

Down Dog

Stretch the palms, chest, back, hamstrings, calves, and feet; strengthen the arms, legs, and torso; and energize the entire body with Down Dog. Improve focus and willpower, stimulate the mind, reduce stress, and relieve low back pain. If you're just beginning, you may find this pose to be challenging, as it does require upper body stamina. Modify by using a chair until you can build up strength.

3. On an inhalation, lift your hips and lengthen through your spine as you roll your shoulders open.

4. Exhale and step back a little more, taking the stretch deeper.

5. Continue to deepen into the pose with every breath, making adjustments and letting your body begin to blossom open.

6. Then bend one knee as you gently press your opposite heel into the floor. Switch legs. Continue to alternate legs, moving into a "bicycle" motion. Repeat five or six reps on each side, then press back into modified Down Dog.

7. Hold for three to ten breaths, then bend both knees and walk your feet forward.

8. Draw your navel in and let go of the chair as you roll back up to standing.

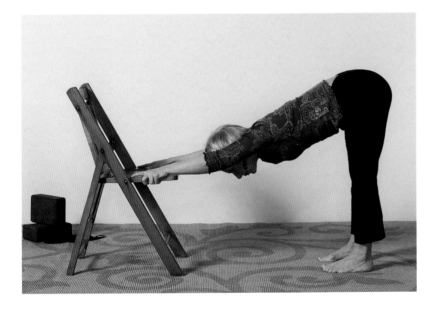

1. Place a sturdy chair in front of you—the seat should be facing you. Place your hands at the edges of the seat and hold on.

2. Begin to step back with your right foot and then your left, until you can extend your spine completely. Breathe into the stretch, inhaling and exhaling deeply.

Bridge

Bridge pose will awaken your spine and open up your belly, releasing tight abdominal muscles. It improves flexibility in the shoulders and spine; stimulates the thyroid and parathyroid glands; increases lung capacity; and relieves high blood pressure, stress, and asthma. Holding Bridge when you're a beginner, or if you have back pain, can be difficult, but you can still reap all the benefits by modifying the pose by using a block.

1. Bend your knees and place your feet flat on the floor, parallel and hips' width apart. Rest your arms alongside your body, with your palms flat.

2. Scoop your tailbone forward and rest your low back as close to the floor as is comfortable. Pull your navel in, keeping your core center strong.

3. On an inhalation, press into the soles of your feet and lift your hips up. Use your glutes to help lift.

4. Feel the weight of your body shifting toward your shoulders, then take your block and place it directly under your sacrum (low back). Let your low body rest on the block and let your arms rest alongside your body.

5. Hold for three to ten breaths, then remove the block, draw your navel in, and slowly lower, tucking your pelvis as you roll through each vertebra.

6. As soon as your tailbone touches the floor, let your knees fall open, place the soles of your feet together, and rest.

7. Bring your knees back together and hug them into your chest, then go into the next move.

Plow

Strengthen the spine, stretch the shoulders, stimulate the thyroid and parathyroid glands, relieve backache, and calm the mind with Plow. Just be sure to keep the head and neck in alignment and don't turn your head. If your neck and shoulders are very tight or you have tight hamstrings, you can use a block to modify.

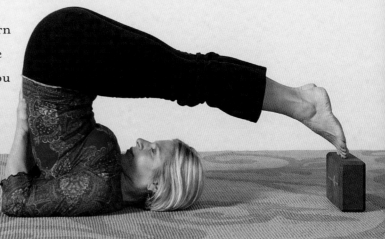

1. Place a block about 12 inches above your head. Lie on your back with your knees pulled into your chest and your hands cradling your hips.

2. Inhale and lift your hips up; then exhale and extend your legs overhead.

3. Keep your hands on your back for support and let your toes rest on the block.

4. Breathe into the pose. Feel your neck elongate as you reach through the crown of your head. Melt your shoulders into the floor and feel the warmth of your breath moving into your cervical spine.

5. Hold for three to five breaths, then slowly roll down out of the pose.

6. As soon as your tailbone touches the floor, let your knees fall open, place the soles of your feet together, and rest.

7. Bring your knees back together and extend your legs along the floor; then go into the next move.

Chest Expansion

To open up the chest and stretch the muscles of the shoulder and arms. Use a strap if your shoulders are very tight.

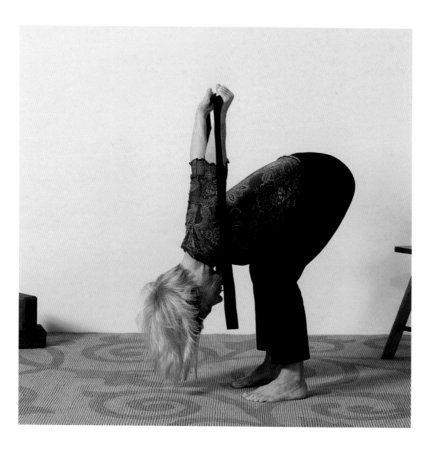

1. Hold the strap in one hand (closer to the middle than the end). Sweep your arms behind your back and grab hold of the strap with the other hand.

2. Slide your hands toward each other, stopping when you feel your shoulders begin to stretch.

3. Exhale and extend your tailbone up to the ceiling, letting your arms fall overhead, surrendering to gravity and your breath.

4. Hold for three to five breaths, then pull your navel in and extend out through the crown of your head. Keep a flat back and let your arms pull you back up.

Fish

A wonderfully restorative pose, Fish strengthens the muscles of the upper back, neck, and shoulders; helps relieve asthma and stress; improves your voice, digestion, and posture; and energizes the mind.

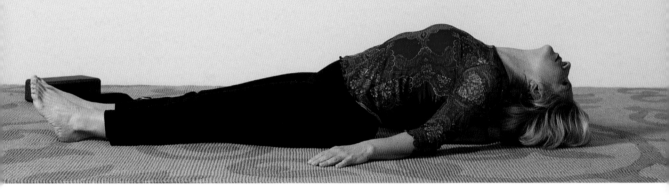

1. Extend your legs along the floor and bring them together, as if they were tied or glued together.

2. Place the block on the floor lengthwise and flat. Lie down with the block under your upper back.

3. Roll your hips from side to side and slide your arms underneath your body. Make sure that your elbows are under your torso and that you're sitting on your hands, with your palms facing the floor.

4. Inhale, press into your elbows as you lift your chest and let your head drop back. Exhale and release the crown of your head to the floor.

5. Hold for three to ten breaths, letting your lungs expand and your throat open.

6. Remove the block and slowly lower your back down and hug your knees.

7. Drop your feet to the floor, let your knees fall open as you bring the soles of your feet together, and rest.

Standing Forward Fold

Strengthen your feet, knees, and thighs; stretch your hamstrings and calves; improve digestion; open up your hips and groin; and soothe your nervous system while you flush your brain with fresh blood and oxygen. Such a healthful pose, but if you have back problems or are brand new to the practice, you may need to use a block to avoid strain on the back.

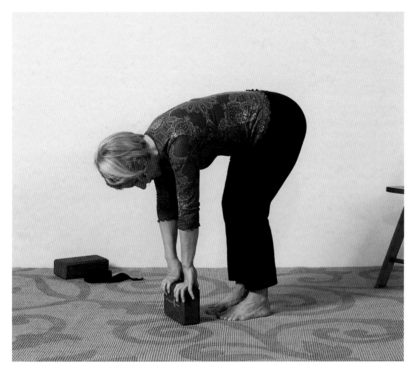

1. Stand with feet hips' width apart, then, keeping a slight bend in your knees to protect your low back, fold forward and place your block right in front of your toes.

(You can turn the block on either end to change the height. As you get more comfortable in the pose, keep adjusting the height until you no longer need to use it.)

2. Bring your awareness into the hinges of your hips and think about elongating and draping your torso over your legs. Release the crown of your head toward the floor.

3. Bend your knees deeply and rest your belly on your thighs. This will free your spine and allow you to release the weight of your upper body. Feel yourself surrendering completely.

4. Breathe deeply, letting go of tension with every exhalation. Shake your head yes and then no to release tension in the cervical spine.

5. Try to stay in Forward Fold for five to ten breaths, continuing to breathe deeply, letting go of the weight of your head and stretching your back.

6. Press through the soles of your feet and draw your navel in as you slowly roll back up to standing.

Triangle

Triangle is also called Happy Pose because it opens up your heart center, allowing you to give and receive joy and love! It also relieves stress and sciatica, which may make you feel happy, too, and it lengthens your spine, stabilizes your torso and your legs, and builds focus. You may find your upper body caves forward as you try to rest your hand on your leg or the floor. But remember, your body should be moving laterally, and you can help make this happen by using a block.

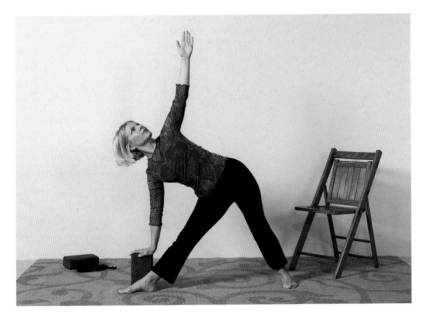

1. Standing with your feet wide apart and parallel, turn your right toes to the right side and keep your left toes straight or slightly turned in. Place a block to the outside of your right foot.

2. Inhale and extend your arms out to your sides; then turn your head to gaze over the middle finger of your right hand.

3. Engage the muscles in your legs and feel your feet root to the floor. Inhale and extend your right fingertips over your right toes, as if someone were pulling your fingers. Keep the torso long.

4. Exhale as you windmill your arms down, letting your right hand rest on the block.

5. Your body should be moving laterally—imagine being pressed between two panes of glass.

6. Gaze up at your left thumb or, if your neck hurts, look down at your big toe. Breathe deeply—keep making adjustments and notice the changes occurring in your body as you sink deeper into the pose.

7. Hold for three to five breaths; then inhale and let your extended (left) arm pull you back up.

8. Turn your toes in the opposite direction and repeat the sequence to the other side.

Straddle Twist

Believe it or not, the wider your legs are in this pose, the easier it will be. This is a wonderful strengthener for your feet, ankles, knees, inner thighs, and lower back. It will also tone your abdominal muscles, build focus and willpower, reduce stress, and even help relieve sinus problems. To modify the pose, place a block about a foot in front of you, at your center.

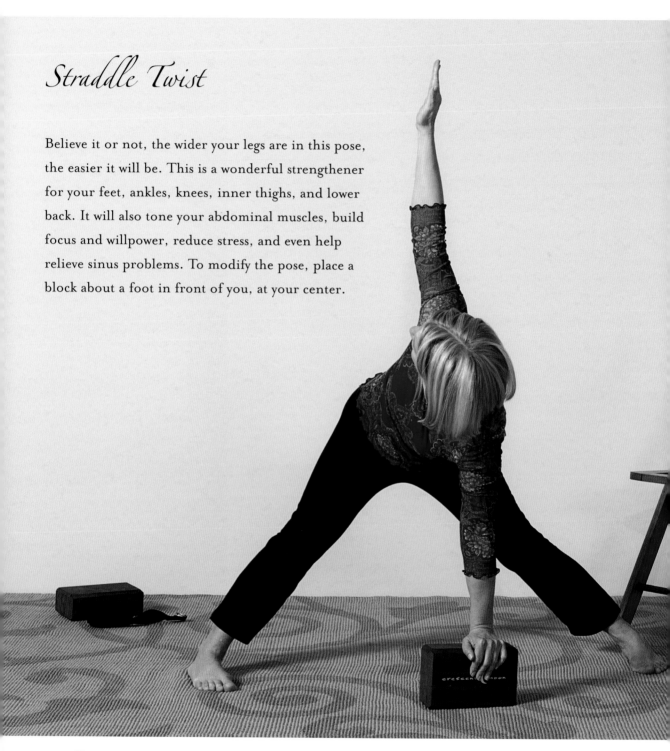

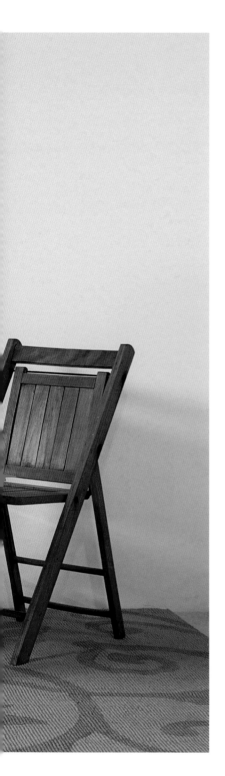

1. Stand with your feet together, arms at your sides, with your palms turned forward. Let your knees face forward and stack them over your ankles. Then stack your hips over your knees, scooping your pelvis forward, and let your tailbone turn downward.

2. Inhale and extend both arms overhead, stretching though your abdominal wall, lifting your rib cage, and sending energy out through all ten fingers.

3. Bend your knees and exhale, letting your arms sweep out to your sides, and float your torso down. Keep the length in your spine as you fold forward.

4. Heel-toe feet apart (anywhere from three to five feet) into a straddle position and keep your feet parallel or your heels a little wider than your toes.

5. Place your hands on the block and keep your spine long and flat. Shift the weight of your body back.

6. Place your left hand on the block and turn your hand so the pinky side faces out.

7. Bring your right hand onto your right hip. Inhale and roll your right shoulder up to the ceiling, turning your entire torso from the hips.

8. Extend your right fingertips up toward the ceiling and gaze up at your thumb.

9. Keep your wrist, elbow, and shoulder of your right arm in one long line. Press into the block and twist your torso deeper.

10. Hold for three to five breaths; then release, come back to center, switch hands, and repeat to the other side.

Using Props Sequence

This is not strictly a sequence, but I did want you to see that you can move from pose to pose even while using props. In fact, many yoga classes will be specifically designated "props classes." Don't think, though, that this means the poses are necessarily easier. In fact, props often allow you to get a deeper stretch or twist than you can reach for on your own. You should feel free to use any of these postures in the other sequences in the book.

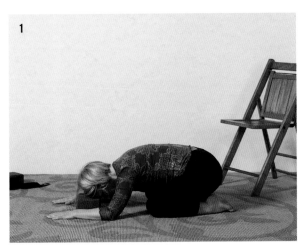

1

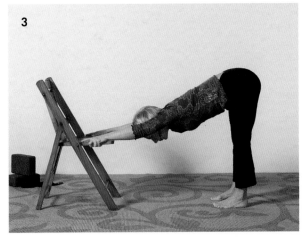

3

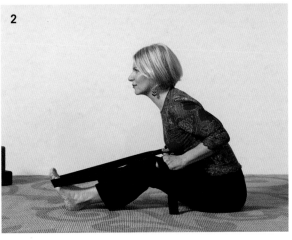

2

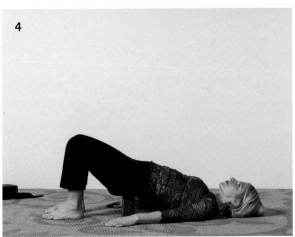

4

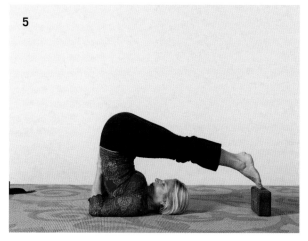

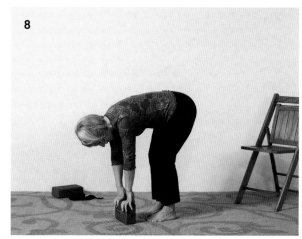

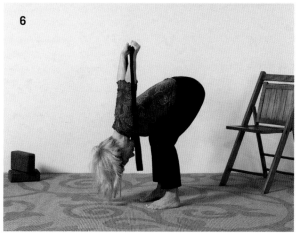

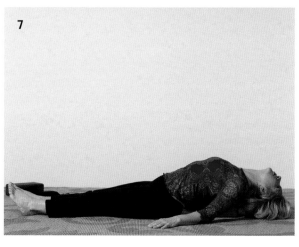

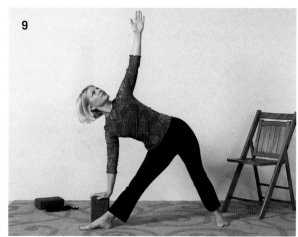

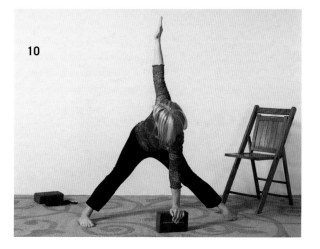

CHAPTER FIFTEEN

Healing Through Meditation

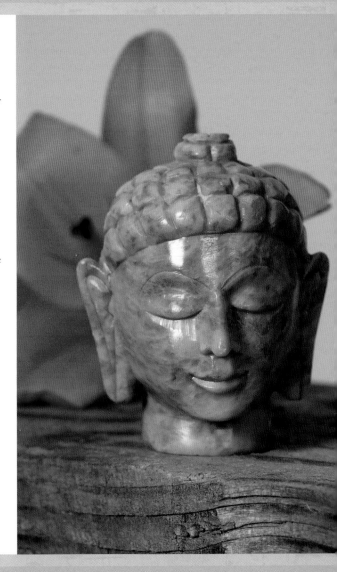

It can be difficult for a doctor

to pin-point the exact cause of a patient's back pain. In fact, mechanical disorders are not the only cause of pain. Depression, anxiety, frustration, stress, anger, and fear, as well as many other negative psychological states, can not only help cause the onset of back or other physical problems, but can also exist as a result of pain.

Whether you are aware of it or not, the body and the mind are in a state of constant interaction. The yogis believe that the body and mind exist as an integrated entity and that the turmoil of daily life brings stress to the body and to the mind, creating anxiety, depression, restlessness, and rage.

In the Yoga Sutras, the great sage Patanjali attributed the causes of mental afflictions to the ego, spiritual ignorance, desire, hatred of others, and attachment to life. He called these *kleshas*, or sorrows. And that was 6,000 years ago—imagine what he would have to say about our modern situations!

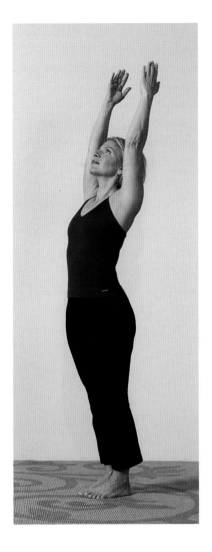

Meditation in Motion

In today's world, emotional distress, financial burdens, and a sense of being overtaken by the speed of modern events have increased stress levels in our daily lives tenfold. These factors strain the body and cause extreme nervous tension. For some, feelings of isolation and loneliness set in. Many people try to deal with this rollercoaster ride by turning to artificial solutions such as drugs, eating disorders, or destructive relationships. While these things may temporarily alleviate stress, or distract the mind, for the most part, the root of the stress stays unresolved.

In order to deal with the strains of life, we draw on our vital life force or energy reserves from our storehouse—the nerve cells. When energy reserves become exhausted due to stress overload, it can lead to the collapse of mental and physical balance.

Yoga is not a miracle cure, but it can help minimize stress. Yoga postures, although appearing to deal with only the physical body, actually influence the chemical balance of the brain, which, in turn, improves one's mental state.

Yoga science teaches that the nerves control the unconscious mind, so when the nervous system is strong, a person can more positively cope with stressful situations. Asana practice helps to improve blood flow to all of the cells of the body and especially helps to revitalize nerve cells. This flow strengthens the nervous system and its capacity for enduring stress.

Journey to the Center of Yourself

In recent years, it has become generally accepted that many physical disorders are not the result of physical breakdown alone—many are rooted in the mind and are a direct cause of stress.

There are two kinds of stress: chronic and acute. Chronic stress happens over time and can be the result of something like a bad relationship or money woes. On the other hand, a sudden occurrence such as an accident or losing your job can bring on acute stress. But no matter which kind of stress we're subjected to, our bodies respond with a natural reaction called flight-or-flight. It's a reaction that can be easily observed in the animal world. When an animal is threatened, it has two choices: stand up and fight or run for its life. How the animal deals with the stress is a result of an instant judgment call: Is the danger life threatening? Is fighting worth the risk? Can the animal get away quickly?

Although human beings generally no longer have to worry about surviving in the wild, our daily stressful dilemmas result in the same kind of primal reaction. Long hours on the job, family crisis, and ongoing world problems can feel like constant attacks. When our fight-or-flight response kicks in, stress hormones like adrenaline and cortisol are released into the body's system, causing muscles to become tense, sensory perception to heighten, and the heart to beat faster. Blood is diverted away from the gastrointestinal system and toward muscles to enable you to perform a physical action. Your pupils dilate so you can see better, your hair stands on end, your skin becomes more sensitive, and your breath rate increases so that more oxygen can be delivered to your body.

Once in a while, this kind of reaction can be a big help, especially if there's a task that needs to be completed—your senses will be sharper and your reaction time quicker—but if your stress level is always turned up high, the autonomic nervous system can become overtaxed. The result includes chronic muscle tension such as tightness in the neck and shoulders, a clenched jaw, sleeplessness, and problems with digestion, to name but a few. It may even cause you to become exhausted and unable to concentrate or communicate effectively. Eventually, this high-stress lifestyle will manifest in a decreased vitality level and overall poor health.

Keep in mind that all this aggravation and stress gets stored in your body, causing blockages, pain, and chemical imbalance. Clearing these blockages and restoring the flow of life force must be accomplished in order for the self-healing process to begin.

Meditation is a wonderful way to begin to heal the body/mind because it helps put us back in touch with all of the sensations, both physical and emotional, which help us get a clearer perspective on life. That's not to say that it's a magic elixir—it can't cure infection or mend broken bones—but meditation can definitely help remove all those obstacles we love to attach ourselves to.

Meditation 101

Most people in today's world can understand and accept that an unsettled state of mind can greatly influence the chemical balance and the physical functioning of the body. If your mind is disturbed by a constant flow of negative feelings, it causes an imbalance in the entire body that some refer to as a state of dis-ease. Worry, anxiety, and resentment can also restrict the flow of vital energy, which shows up as physical symptoms and can be as damaging to our bodies as any chemical toxin. Meditation has been proven to be highly effective in treating the source of these psychic disturbances by bringing balance back to the body.

Ailments such as migraine headaches, anxiety attacks, sinus problems, asthma, and cardiac arrhythmias can also be helped by the regular deep breathing exercises included in meditation practice, which help to increase air flow through constricted passages. In addition, regular practice and relaxation techniques lower levels of stress hormones in the body while improving self-discipline and sports performance, building confidence, increasing energy and efficiency, and creating a more positive outlook. And positive people, we all know, get sick less often and generally live longer and happier lives.

Meditation also helps regulate blood pressure, stimulates circulation, alleviates pain, and reduces muscular tension. It's not hard to spot people who practice regularly—they just look better and more fit.

Everybody's Doing It

Ten million American adults say they practice some form of meditation, and more and more doctors recommend it as a way to prevent or at least control the pain of chronic diseases such as heart conditions, cancer, and infertility. Meditation also helps restore balance to those suffering from depression, hyperactivity, or attention deficit disorder (ADD). And after years of research, scientific studies are now beginning to show that it really does work.

In the 1960s, Professor Robert Wallace of the University of California and Dr. Herbert Benson, a Harvard cardiologist, confirmed studies that proved meditation has a profound physiological effect on the body—more than just sleeping or simply relaxing. When you are in a meditative state, you inhale 17 percent less oxygen and 17 percent less carbon dioxide than in conventional relaxation techniques. Blood pressure and heart rate are significantly less, and lactic acid remains at a low level for a long time after practicing. (Lactic acid is an indicator of stress levels and is associated with the flight-or-fight response.) A few years later, Harvard psychiatry professor Dr. Gregg Jacobs proved that meditation helps produce more theta waves in the brain—the kind of waves that dominate the brain during periods of deep relaxation.

During the same period, two Japanese researchers concurred, proving that during meditation, the brain patterns of Zen monks corresponded to the low theta frequency usually associated with sleep even though the monks were wide awake and, in fact, in a heightened state of awareness. It was also discovered that regular meditation could be used to control physiological functions such as heart rate and body temperature, which eventually led to the development of biofeedback—the alternative method that uses ancient meditation techniques to help patients learn to relieve pain and stress.

Easing Pain

Living with pain, especially chronic back pain, can overtake your life. Almost every decision you make on any given day depends on how bad the pain is at that time. The stress can be overwhelming, and as a result, life becomes difficult.

Meditation practice can help you to deal with debilitating back pain in many ways. Try this simple technique: Lie down on your back and make yourself comfortable. You might want to place a pillow or blanket underneath your knees to relieve stress on the low back, or you could place a small pillow under your head and neck.

Close your eyes and focus on your breath for a few moments until you start to feel more relaxed. Slowly let your awareness move into your body and acknowledge the area that is experiencing pain. Try to watch the pain as if you were an outside observer. Begin to give the pain shape and color. Allow the color to become brighter or deeper in hue, and then allow the shape to change. If the pain lessens or becomes more intense, imagine the shape and color changing along with it. As you continue to watch the pain, imagine it floating out of your body and hanging outside of you so that you can see it more easily. Do not let your mind get involved with the pain, but do explore it and become acquainted with it. Practice this visualization for a few days, and then start to consciously change the shape and color of the pain. It may take some time, but you may be able to achieve some control over the pain and eventually learn to form some kind of manageable relationship with it.

Breath

According to yogis, the diaphragm is the seat of the intelligence of the heart and the window to the soul. However, when you're stressed, inhaling and exhaling become difficult because the diaphragm becomes too taut to alter its shape. Yoga postures develop elasticity in the diaphragm, so that when you're stressed—whether emotionally, physically, or intellectually—you'll be able to handle it.

Practicing yoga, breath, and meditation helps to integrate the body, mind, and intellect. The slow exhalations that are practiced during asana work help to bring serenity to the body cells; to relax the facial muscles; and to release tension from the eyes, ears, nose, tongue, and skin. When this happens, the brain—which is in constant communication with the organs—becomes still and all thoughts are released.

Alternate Nostril Breathing

This is one of my favorite breathing techniques because it helps to bring both physical and emotional balance to the body/mind. It's especially great after a long day or if you just need to clear the brain and get focused.

- Begin in a seated position, making sure your spine is erect but comfortable.

- Let your left hand rest lightly on your left thigh and bring your right hand in front of your face.

- Fold down your index and middle finger, leaving your thumb extended and your ring and pinky fingers extended.

- Cover your right nostril with your thumb and draw in a deep breath through your left nostril.

- Close off your left nostril with your ring and pinky fingers and release your thumb as you breathe out through your right nostril.

- Inhale through your right, then close it off.

- Exhale through your left.

- Inhale through your left; close it off.

- Exhale through your right.

- Continue on, alternating for as little as one minute or for as long as five, until you feel yourself becoming more centered and calm.

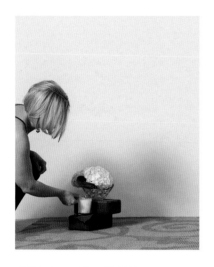

Enlightened Paths

There are many ways to meditate, some are purely spiritual and some involve a more physical practice. It's helpful to try a few to see which one suits your personality and situation best.

Concentrative

This is a meditative technique that helps focus the mind on a particular point such as the breath, a candle flame, or a mandala (a circular geometric design that draws the eye to its center). Meditating with open eyes will keep you grounded and also make you less likely to fall asleep. It can help keep distractions—even imaginary ones—away from your line of vision.

Candle Gazing or Trataka

Candle gazing may be performed at any time on an empty stomach. Ten minutes a day is all you'll need, but you can vary the time depending on your specific needs. Beginners can start with shorter periods of time and build up.

Begin by setting a candle about one to two feet away from you. Sit in a comfortable position and take a few deep breaths. Then bring your hands to prayer position at your heart center and gently rub your palms together. Press your warm palms into your eyes and allow the heat to penetrate, melting soreness and redness. Keep them there until the heat dissipates, then begin.

- Continuously gaze at the flame and try not to blink.

- Allow your gaze to remain smooth and effortless.

- Stay focused; use your willpower and try to ignore watering in the eyes.

- Hold your gaze for thirty to sixty seconds.

- Bring your palms back onto the eyes and rest for thirty seconds.

- Focus on the whole flame for a few moments.

- Now focus intently on the tip of the wick.

- Focus on the whole flame for a few seconds.

- Slowly soften your focus as you defocus your attention.

- Palm the eyes: press them gently, then release.

- Expand your vision and begin to notice the aura around the flame.

- Watch it gradually becoming bigger and bigger.

- Observe the tiny light particles around the flame.

- Now bring your focus back onto the whole flame.

- Close your eyes and visualize the afterimage of the flame.

- As the image fades, bring your palms to your eyes.

Mindfulness

Simply put, mindfulness means letting go and accepting that you cannot control your thoughts—so that you can stop letting thoughts control you. Try to observe your thoughts with detachment—as if you were watching images play across the screen of your mind. Don't attach any emotions or judgments to the thoughts, and try not to give them a significance they don't deserve. Remember that we live only in the present moment—the past is over, it's part of our history, we can't change it. The future is imaginary. We have no control over the future, no way of knowing what it will bring, so why try to figure it out? Mindful meditation is about the reality of being present, and it is, in fact, the true nature of our consciousness.

Mindful Moments

As you go about your daily routine, stop from time to time and notice the state of your awareness. Are you completely paying attention to what you're doing, or are you distracted and tense and worried about the next task? Take a deep breath and hold it for two or three counts, then exhale very slowly. Bring your awareness into the present moment, then continue with what you were doing but remain mindful of the moment at hand.

BE AWARE

Sitting in a comfortable position, bring your attention to your breath and close your eyes. When you feel relaxed, begin to notice sounds in the room, then bring the awareness into your body. Notice the sensation of your sitting bones resting on the floor, the heaviness of your bones and muscles. Then notice the air on your skin and the way your clothing feels on your body. Observe if you're feeling warm or cool. Now bring the awareness to your inner body; notice if there are any muscle contractions or rumblings in your digestive tract. Come back to your breath and notice the coolness of the inhales and the warmth of the exhales. Slowly allow yourself to become aware of what's going on in your mind. Let thoughts and images play across the screen of your mind. Notice feelings and emotions. Don't try to change anything, just be aware. Begin to turn your attention to the awareness itself. Allow yourself to become aware of the knowingness that lets you perceive all of these sensations. Pay attention to the attention and allow yourself to be the awareness.

Your World in Review

Here's a useful visualization to help you sleep. Close your eyes and focus on your breath for a few moments. Don't try to change it, simply find the rhythm of it and get into the flow. Now begin to review the events of your day, starting with the present moment and going backward until the moment you awoke. Don't linger on any one event or person or conversation, just rerun them and try to recall as much detail as possible. Include as many physical sensations as you can, such as textures, smells, and temperature. Remain detached, with no judgments. Don't allow yourself to take anything personally. When you get to the moment of awakening, let go and visualize a stream of images fast-forwarding on the screen of your mind. Acknowledge that the day is over and is now a part of your history. You can't relive it. Let your intention for tomorrow be that you will live every moment for the present.

Visualization

Clearing away negative conditioning can go a long way to help heal your body and revitalize your life. And visualizations are an effective way to deprogram these negative thoughts and help attract whatever it is that you want. They can also help to bring about personal growth by helping you to better communicate with your higher self. In this technique, imagery and symbols help unlock the unconscious mind, and you can either control the scene or let the events unfold.

Movement

If you practice yoga, you're doing a form of moving meditation. Moving heightens your awareness of physical sensations and something as simple as a walk through a beautiful garden on a spring morning or taking a tai chi class can help soothe and calm your mind and body.

A Walk in the Park

To practice a walking meditation, it's best to find a long, straight path in the country or perhaps on a beach. It should be a favorite place if possible, but even if you live in the city, you can practice meditation by changing the focus of your attention every time you turn onto a new street.

When you begin your walk, acknowledge the wind on your face, the way the earth feels under your feet, the light, the colors, the smells, and the sounds. Try not to attach thought or judgment to the experience; instead, just enjoy the present moment. The object is to be mindful of your surroundings as well as your body. If you become distracted by thoughts, bring yourself back into the moment, back into the state of detached awareness.

Loving Kindness

This practice helps cultivate a positive outlook and mood as well as compassion, forgiveness, and love for all people. (See meditation on facing page.)

Love Really Is All You Need

Come into a comfortable seated position and close your eyes. Begin to watch your breath for a few moments, letting yourself find a rhythm, an ebb and flow, and then feel yourself centering. Begin thinking about a person that you love or have loved and imagine you're with this person. Visualize him or her beside you and pay attention to the details. What is he or she wearing? Where are you? Begin to open up to the feeling of love for this person. Allow your entire mind and body to fill with this joyful love, and then let go of the person. Now begin to focus entirely on the feeling of love, and be present in the feeling of love's energy moving and flowing within your heart and soul.

Transformative

In this type of practice, the meditator can seek a solution to a problem or turn negative emotions into positive energy.

Accept Yourself

As you begin this meditation, keep in mind that before you can become who you truly want to be, you have to learn to accept who you are right now.

Come into a comfortable position. You can be seated or lying down. Close your eyes and focus on your breath until you find a rhythm and become calm and centered. Visualize a cluster of stars in a clear and bright night sky. As you continue to gaze into the infinite darkness, focus on one tiny dot of light in the distance. Continue to gaze at the light, letting it expand and become more intense. Watch the light as it opens up into particles of light and energy, and let this brilliant energy form a pair of hands. In the hands, you notice a happy, smiling baby. The baby is you. It's not the you who has been burdened by worldly concerns or whatever problems you find yourself dealing with over and over again. This is the real you, the universal child who cannot die. Pain, loneliness, disappointment, fear, anger, and all other negative emotions have no meaning to this child. This is a child created from eternal light, whose purpose is to love and be loved. Discover an understanding that, if, for some reason, this love has not been returned, it is no fault of the child's. Understand that the highest purpose and only obligation of the child is to show love in this present moment.

Transcendental Meditation (TM)

Transcendental meditation differs from any traditional forms of meditation in one way: It emphasizes the importance of a mantra, which is personal and kept to oneself. Maharishi Mahesh Yogi (the Beatles' personal guru) brought TM to the West in 1958. It has gained widespread acceptance in the medical community for its ability to help relieve stress, psychosomatic disorders, and addictions.

Sound vibrations and mantras are thought to have a healing effect on the body because they induce a relaxed state that promotes healing. Studies have shown that the repetition of a single word not only slows the heart rate and

Finding a mantra that suits you is not complicated. Some people find chanting their own name to be very effective, while others choose a word in a different language or a word that will help evoke a particular feeling, such as "relax."

Choose a word that best suits you, then get into a comfortable meditative position. Take a deep breath and let the air come out slowly and evenly as you chant your chosen word. Say the word clearly and loudly so that it creates a vibration in your body. Say the word over and over and try to create a continuous sound so that each repetition melts into the next. Get into a flowing rhythm and allow yourself to become mesmerized by the sound. Gradually you can reduce the volume until it is created only in your mind. Eventually let it disappear altogether, and let yourself exist in stillness.

lowers blood pressure, but also calms the brain by increasing alpha-wave activity, which is associated with drowsiness and relaxed attention.

According to neuroscientists at Moscow's Brain Research Institute in Russia, this form of meditation produces a unique pattern of coherent activity in the brain's frontal cortex, creating a state of "restful alertness" and improved mental performance.

How to Begin

Try to practice twice daily for at least ten minutes at a time, preferably at the same time each day. It's nice to begin your day with a meditation. It helps to clear away the psychic debris left over from the previous day and prepares you to face whatever challenges are in store for you in the coming day. Creating this reflective and safe space provides us with the beautiful gift of quiet time for ourselves, giving us the chance to discover who we truly are and what we truly want out of life. It's a unique opportunity to nurture ourselves, tap into our inner resources, and find a lasting sense of peace. Anyone can mediate, but it will take practice and discipline.

We are constantly bombarded and stimulated with modern life, and we are conditioned to look for a quick fix in food, entertainment, drink, or drugs. Setting aside time to do "nothing" may seem totally self-indulgent, but it's actually just as necessary as physical exercise for overall well-being.

Persevere

Put aside all those things that seem more worthwhile than meditating. Trust me—this is one of the most important things you'll do for yourself!

Remember that when you begin a new exercise program, you need a certain amount of self-discipline and practice. You may not know the proper form for a military press or a triceps kickback, but eventually, with enough practice, you learn and become more aware of your physical body. Each time you get into the gym, your form gets better and your muscles get bigger. It's the same with meditation. When you first begin, it will be difficult to keep distractions from your mind: Did you feed the cat? What time is that meeting tomorrow? Why is my foot itchy? Don't worry. Anyone who meditates will tell you that it's common to feel frustrated and distracted when you're first starting out. Once you begin to feel the benefits, it will get easier and you'll be hooked.

You might want to have a focus or an intention each time you practice. Cultivate compassion by sending out a healing energy to someone who is in need. It will help you to become less self-centered.

Relax

Reaching a relaxed state is not as easy as you might think. Most of us have become addicted to the chemical high that comes from the constant motion of life. When we do take a moment to slow down, it's usually in an unfocused way and may actually end up causing more stress (think traveling, overeating, drinking). Contemplation and quiet reflection require mindfulness in order to be successful.

Music for Meditation

Music is a wonderful tool that provides focus and helps to quiet the mind. In Eastern cultures, bells or drums or single sustained notes are part of the meditation ritual. Recent studies suggest that instrumental music that maintains a constant tempo of sixty beats per minute can induce the alpha state (a relaxed sense of alertness where the brain can more easily retain information) and help to reprogram the mind with positive suggestions to promote healing and help achieve goals.

Resources

Austin, Miriam. *Cool Yoga Tricks.* New York: Ballantine Books, 2003.

Blahnik, Jay. *Full-Body Flexibility.* Champaign, IL: Human Kinetics, 2004.

Borenstein, David, MD. *Back in Control.* New York: M. Evans and Company, Inc., 2001.

Earle, Roger E., and Thomas Baechle. *NSCA's Essentials of Personal Training.* Champaign, IL: Human Kinetics, 2003.

Fitness Theory and Practice, 2nd ed. Aerobics and Fitness Association of America, 1995.

Iyengar, BKS. *Yoga: The Path to Holistic Health.* New York: DK Publishing, 2001.

Kirk, Martin, and Brooke Boon, *Hatha Yoga Illustrated.* Champaign, IL: Human Kinetics, 2004.

Payne, Larry, Ph.D., and Richard Usatine, MD, *Yoga Rx.* New York: Broadway Books, 2001.

Robinson, Lynn, Helge Fisher, and Paul Massey. *The Pilates Prescription for Back Pain.* Berkeley: Ulysses Press, 2004.

Rush Presbyterian-St. Luke's Medical Center. *Medical Encyclopedia.* Chicago: World Book Publishing, 1999.

Sarno, John E., MD. *Healing Back Pain.* New York: Warner Books, 1991.

Scott, Judith. *Goodbye to Bad Backs.* Hightstown, NJ: Dance Horizons/Princeton Book Company, 1988.

Stanmore, Tia. *The Pilates Back Book.* Gloucester, MA: Fair Winds Press, 2002.

Also

Back.com

Consumer Reports on Health newsletter

DynoMed.com

Acknowledgments

If not for Melissa McNeese (thank you!), I would never have met Donna Raskin, who is not only an incredible editor and writer, but who has become a good friend. Donna's enthusiasm and encouragement during this project provided a buoy of support that I appreciate beyond words.

The staff at Fair Winds was not only fun to work with, but also wonderfully helpful, especially during a few divalike moments at the photo shoot. Special thanks to Allan, Bevan, Silke, Claire, and Rhia for keeping their sense of humor and making me feel completely comfortable.

To the staff at *Fit* and *Fit Yoga* magazines, thank you so much for your continuous hard work and for making my job easy. An extra-special thank you to Irwin for believing in my abilities and giving me such wonderful opportunities.

And to all my family and friends—thank you for putting up with "my book" for way too many months and for helping me shine my light out into the universe.

CLOTHES PROVIDED BY: Lotuswear, Blue Canoe, Prana, and Yoga Force.

YOGA ACCESSORIES PROVIDED BY: Crescent Moon.

About the Author

Rita Trieger is the editor-in-chief of *Fit* and *Fit Yoga* magazines. She has been practicing yoga and meditation for 20 years, studying at Integral Yoga, Mandali Yoga, Jivamukti, Kundalini East and Bikram. She has participated in workshops and trained with some of the yoga world's most respected teachers, including Baron Baptiste and Rodney Yee, as well as the great meditation teacher, Sally Kempton (formerly Swami Durgananda).

Besides teaching yoga and meditation at The Health and Fitness Institute at Stamford Hospital, Rita teaches for several corporations, as well as World Gym in her native New York, and A WomanSpace, a yoga and pilates studio also in New York.

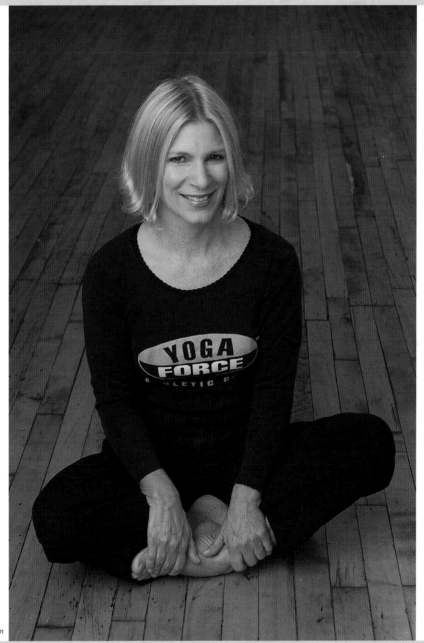

Photo By Tom Carson